NEW VET JUMPSTART GUIDE GP BOOK

SECOND EDITION

YOUR DAY-ONE GUIDE TO
20 GENERAL PRACTICE CASES

Ashley Gray, DVM and
Monica Tarantino, DVM

VETS ON THE RISE

FOR STUDENTS & NEW GRAD VETS

AF703653

New Vet Jumpstart Guide GP Book:
Your Day-One Guide to 20 General Practice Cases

Second Edition

Copyright © 2026 by
Vets on the Rise / Ashley Gray, DVM and Monica Tarantino, DVM

All rights reserved. No portion of this book may be reproduced, stored in a retrieval system, or transmitted in any form or means such as electronic, mechanical, photocopying, recording, or otherwise, without the prior written consent of the author. Small portions may be quoted in a journal, article, or media post.

ISBN: 979-8-218-93450-7 (print)
ISBN: 979-8-218-93451-4 (eBook)

Published by:
Vets on the Rise
Charlotte, North Carolina

VETS ON THE RISE

FOR STUDENTS & NEW GRAD VETS

Hi New Vets! (and welcome back to those returning for round two!)

We are SO pumped to share this second edition of our *New Vet Jumpstart Guide GP Book*. This update means a lot to us, and not just because we have refined and expanded our content, but because we had the incredible opportunity to collaborate with two veterinary specialists we deeply admire: Dr. Jessica Romine (DACVIM) and Dr. Jeff Tinsley (DACVD). They took the time to review the bulk of our work, offer great insights, and helped us level up this book...and we learned so much in the process too!

That right there is the beauty of medicine: it is never static. Things change. Our understanding deepens. New techniques emerge. Staying curious, going to CE, learning from others...it's all part of growing as a vet and as a person. And that's exactly what this book is about: learning, evolving, and becoming more confident in your everyday cases.

As with the first edition, we have focused on the kinds of cases that can trip up even the smartest new grad, and not because you don't care or aren't capable, but because you are still figuring out how to slow down, simplify, and stay grounded when things feel chaotic. We have all been there. This book is about helping you find clarity and direction when it counts most.

Before you dive in, here are some timeless reminders:

- Nothing replaces a thorough physical exam.
- Communication is everything. Most complaints come from *how* things were said or not said at all.
- Talk about the disease process and treatment plan *before* you present the estimate. Once money enters the convo, you often lose your client's focus.
- Don't panic if the answer isn't obvious. Take a breath, be methodical, and use your diagnostics to guide you.
- Be honest. Always. People trust transparency.

- And if your patient isn't responding, first make sure the owner is following the plan (yep, people go rogue). If your initial approach doesn't work, *then* start hunting for zebras. This book is all about starting with the horses.

We are thrilled to have you here with us, whether this is your first read or you are back for the update. Let's keep learning and rising together.

Your Vet Med Besties,
Ashley and Monica
VETS ON THE RISE co-founders

DISCLAIMER STATEMENT

The information contained in this book is provided for educational and informational purposes only and is not intended as, and should not be relied upon as, medical advice, diagnosis, or treatment. This book does not establish a practitioner–patient relationship between the reader and the authors.

The content reflects the authors' clinical experience, professional opinions, and interpretation of available medical research at the time of publication. Some viewpoints, interpretations, or approaches discussed may differ from mainstream medical opinion. Portions of this book reference, summarize, or paraphrase findings from external medical studies, publications, and online sources; such material is cited for informational purposes only and does not imply endorsement or replacement of individualized professional medical judgment.

Medical knowledge and best practices evolve continually. While every effort has been made to ensure the accuracy and relevance of the information presented at the time of writing, the authors, contributors, and editors make no representations or warranties regarding completeness, accuracy, or current applicability of the content.

Readers are strongly advised to consult a qualified healthcare professional before making any medical decisions, including but not limited to the use, dosage, modification, or discontinuation of any medication, supplement, or treatment discussed in this book. Any medication, dosage, or therapeutic approach mentioned should be independently verified with authoritative and up-to-date sources.

The use of any information contained in this book is entirely at the reader's own risk. The authors, editors, contributors, and publishers expressly disclaim any and all liability for injury, illness, death, adverse outcomes, or damage to persons, animals, or property resulting from the use or misuse of the information presented herein.

We want to give a big thank you to the amazing veterinarians who supported and advised us during the creation of our first book collaboration. We had such a great time putting it together for our VOTR family and remain deeply grateful for their encouragement and expertise.

Thank you to:
Angela Gamboni, DVM · Brent Gordon, DVM · Elizabeth Franklin, DVM ·
Jordan Jaeger, DVM, DACVIM (Small Animal Internal Medicine) · Nikki Johnson, DVM ·
Katie Miller, DVM · Julie Reck, DVM · Fred Wininger, DVM, DACVIM (Neurology)

As we release this updated second edition,
we're especially grateful to our brilliant editors and contributors:

Jessica Romine, DVM, DACVIM

Jeff Tinsley, DVM, DACVD

Gabriella Varcoe, DVM, DACVSMR, CCRP

Marie Dantio, DVM, DACVIM

We learned so much from all of you and cannot thank you enough for taking the time to help veterinarians across the world learn from your expert insights.

We are also excited to share our brand-new cover, voted on by you, with a drawing of a photo featuring **Monique Fletcher, DVM.** Thank you to Hayley and Katty for bringing this vision to life with the cover art.

CONTENTS

Advice We Kept Referencing as New Grads

Vaccine reaction or anaphylaxis plan:

- **Mild:** Diphenhydramine 2.2 mg/kg IM or SQ (NOT IV!) +/- DexSP 0.1 mg/kg IV or IM (falling out of favor, but we are still tending to use for brachycephalic breeds or dogs with swelling that could impact their ability to breathe)
  - Monitor your patient for 20-30 minutes to assess response and make sure vitals are stable and symptoms appear to be stabilizing
  - Have pet owner continue diphenhydramine orally for 3-5 days since symptoms can be unpredictable
- **Moderate:** Go between mild and severe based on response to therapy and vital parameters (if trending towards shock, better to be aggressive with a dose of epinephrine too!)
- **Severe:** Get an IV catheter in → give Diphenhydramine 2.2 mg/kg IM or SQ q8 hr, Epinephrine 0.01 mg/kg IM (can be repeated every 5-15 minutes as needed since it does not last long), and Famotidine 0.5-1 mg/kg IM or SQ +/- DexSP 0.1 mg/kg IV or IM (see above under mild for reasoning and more info)
  - Once the catheter is placed, begin additional treatment for shock. Start bolusing fluids **(5-10 mL/kg is the current recommendation for a bolus**, allowing ability to give 2-3 additional if needed...better tailored response to therapy to avoid fluid overload), begin flow-by oxygen, monitor vital parameters, vasopressors or hetastarch if needed (if boluses are not helping...we usually reach for these after 2-3 boluses with pressors superior if you have them in hospital)

IV fluid bolus updates:

- We are going to sound old here by saying this, but "when we were in school..." but yea, we were taught a bolus was ¼-⅓ shock dose so you will see that dose periodically in our books. Now, fluids are being treated more like a 'dose of a medication' because it is hard to take it back if you accidentally overload your patient. The recommended amount we have been doing as of 2026 updates is **5-10 mL/kg IV over 5-15 mins** pending how ill the patient is (a.k.a. slam it in vs. set a pump). We will repeat it up to 1-2 more times if needed while performing diagnostics. By the second-third if we are still not seeing great results (after some diagnostics have been performed to gain more insight), we will then reach for other therapies like blood products, hypertonic saline, or vasopressors.

How to make 2.5% dextrose solution:

- Remove 50 mL of fluid from 1 L bag
- Then, add 50 mL of 50% Dextrose to 1 L bag

To get from % to mg/mL:

- Add a 0 to the %
  - Lasix 5% = 50 mg/mL
  - Dextrose 50% = 500 mg/mL
  - Cosyntropin 1 mg = 1000 mcg

CRI calculation:

- 1: Calculate the fluid rate
- 2: Calculate the # of hours in that bag
- 3: Calculate the dose/hr
- 4: Multiply the # of hours in bag x dose/hr
- 5: Convert to mLs=how many mLs to add to bag (and remove from bag)

Note from Dr. Jess on CRI's (Internal Medicine specialist): At our hospital, we calculate most additives (KCl, metoclopramide, other CRIs we expect an animal to be on for a while) on a 24 mL/hr basis to keep things simple. This strategy allows you to evaluate dosages regularly so that when a syringe runs out, you can decide if you want to continue or not.

- Essentially, figure out the dose per 24 hours, convert to mLs, and add as much saline as needed to create 24 mLs of solution and run at 1 mL/hr (increase or decrease to adjust dose from there).
- This means you can kind of ignore calculating total fluid administration and can adjust fluid rates without worrying about making up new bags with new KCl, metoclopramide, etc.

- Example: 15 kg dog needing metoclopramide CRI for ongoing regurgitation.
    - We start at 2 mg/kg/day: 15 kg x 2 mg/kg/day = 30 mg/day
    - Metoclopramide is 5 mg/mL so that's 6 mL needed per day
    - 24 mL total for a 24 hour CRI: 6 mL metoclopramide + add 18 mL saline to create 24 mL total volume and start at 1 mL/hr
    - Double check that 0.9% saline is okay to use (or sterile water, 5% dextrose, etc. if indicated)

PU/PD:

- Polydipsia is drinking > 100 mL/kg/day
- Polyuria means urinating > 50 mL/kg/day

Other random tidbits:

- Only use DexSP in cats because dexamethasone is glycol based, which is toxic to them.
- Do not forget your PO drugs that can cause esophageal strictures in cats (like doxycycline, clindamycin, etc.). We always recommend chasing pills with 3-5 mL of water after to be safe.
- You cannot ask an owner to split pills into 1/8 or 3/4. It is difficult and reduces compliance. Get it compounded instead.
- Always check for any adverse drug interactions in Plumb's when you have a pet on multiple drugs.
- Mention common medication side effects to owners.
    - Example: We have each had a case where a dog became temporarily deaf from Mometamax usage. Warning an owner of side effects allows them to monitor better, discontinue the drug, and call you right away.
- Famotidine, maropitant, and cefovecin all calculate out to the same amount (0.045 mL/lb).
- Always explain (or utilize your tech) how to give medications clearly. You will be surprised how many people do not know how to give it or do not know strategies to ensure their pet takes the medication.
    - Give them food options to hide pills in like peanut butter, chicken, tuna, wet food (roll it into a meatball), marshmallows, cheese, Pill Pockets/Pill Wrap, etc.

    - ▽ Tell an owner if a medication is bitter (like metronidazole), so they know to hide it well.
    - ▽ Same goes for eye and ear medications. Show them exactly how to administer it by doing the first treatment.

How Dr. Jess approaches the "feed a bland diet" conversation:

Saying feed boiled chicken and white rice only is actually doing a disservice to our patients because they need fiber to help them turn it around efficiently (and without metro!). It will definitely help when coupled with your other diarrhea therapies these days like probiotics (we like Fortiflora and Proviable-kit is great!) and Endosorb.

- ▶ Here is her example conversation to help you:
    - ▽ "Right now, what matters most is that Fluffy is eating enough calories regularly. We don't think this was caused by her normal diet, so if she is eating that, I'm okay with her going back to it, but if she's not up for it yet, we're going to be offering her highly digestible, nutrient-dense foods. The three main commercial options are Hill's I/D, Royal Canin Gastrointestinal, and Purina EN. All come in wet and dry forms, and I'm okay with any of the formulations. If she needs to be tempted with human food, always cook it as her gut cannot process bacteria in raw food right now. She can be offered lean meat (chicken breast with no skin, turkey, drained lean beef mince, white fish, etc), low-fat cottage cheese, yogurt, pasta, potatoes, sweet potatoes, and rice."
    - ▽ "It's important to know that while all of these above foods are nice and easy to digest, they have almost no fiber, and this can lead to diarrhea and difficulty regaining colon health. So an easy thing to do if Fluffy is still having loose stools is to add in some fiber, such as Fiber One cereal (ensure no raisins!). Most dogs don't mind the taste, and it can get mixed right in with the food."
        - ➔ **Her dose for fiber (Fiber One cereal or equivalent product):** For <5 kg dog/cat, I start at 1 teaspoon twice daily, 5-15 kg 1/2 tablespoon, >15 kg 1 tablespoon. If needed, you can increase by the same volume every 2-3 days up to 4x start (4 teaspoons, 2 tablespoons, 4 tablespoons twice daily respectively). Don't go too high too fast as too much fiber can loosen stools

too. Owners usually love the idea and it's amazing how many respond. We all need more fiber in our diets, people and dogs!

- **Other fiber options?:** Psyllium is usually ¼ to ½ teaspoon per 10 kg and can work up to 1-2 teaspoons/10 kg, but work up slowly. Most nutritionists don't use Metamucil. They use NOW brand or Konsyl because they are not cut with flavorings. Wagtritious, Profibre and Proviable Fiber powder are also good products to consider.

- Hill's GI Biome and RC Fiber Response can be awesome mix-ins here too!
- **NOTE:** unless a dog has proven actual recurrent pancreatitis or hypertriglyceridemia, they don't need to be put on low-fat food, particularly if the upset was induced by them eating something they shouldn't. Avoid high fat, but they don't need low-fat food for life.

NOTES:

NOTES:

NOTES:

Chronic Diarrhea in Older Cats

Reviewed by Dr. Jessica Romine, DVM, DACVIM

When a cat presents to you with chronic diarrhea, you will often find a frustrated owner in the exam room. As you know, there are many differentials that can cause chronic diarrhea, so a work-up is needed. When working these patients up, the most important thing you can do is to progress in a methodical manner ruling conditions out in a step by step fashion. You do not want to get burned by parasites, so start simple with fecal testing and deworming, even in an indoor only cat. The basic diagnostic plan we lay out here will get you far.

The second most important thing you need to do with these cases is communicate clearly with the client. Let them know upfront that these cases can be frustrating. Then, let them know the initial course of action you will take and how you will be working in a methodical step by step manner. We will try one thing first, and if this is ineffective, then we move on to the next diagnostic or treatment plan. Lastly, keep them informed on what the next step of the plan is if the current treatment does not work. This helps owners feel involved and prepared. Let's get started!

Here is our basic approach:

1. Differentiate between small and large intestinal diarrhea
2. Confirm acute or chronic diarrhea is present
3. Diagnostic plan
4. Treatment plan

STEP 1: Differentiate between small and large intestinal diarrhea.

- Getting a good history will guide you.
- Small intestinal: large stool volume, weight loss, changes in appetite, abdominal discomfort, melena, etc.
- Large intestinal: small volume, tenesmus, hematochezia, frequent, etc.

STEP 2: Confirm acute or chronic diarrhea is present.

- Again, history will guide you. Chronic diarrhea typically lasts three weeks or more.

STEP 3: Diagnostic plan:

Common differential list

- Dietary: food allergy, food intolerance, raw diet, etc.
- Exocrine pancreatic insufficiency
- Infection: viral, bacterial, parasitic, fungal, etc.
  - Examples: Salmonella, Campylobacter, Giardia, Coccidia, Cryptosporidium, Tritrichomonas, Felv, FIP, SIBO, etc.
- Infiltrative: lymphoma, other neoplasia
- Inflammatory: inflammatory bowel disease, pancreatitis, cholangitis, cholangiohepatitis, triaditis
- Metabolic/systemic disease: hyperthyroidism, liver disease, kidney disease, etc.

FIP Differential Tidbit from Dr. Jess

At my practice, we have identified multiple older cats with FIP. Their presenting complaints are diarrhea, weight loss, and a really thick ileocolic junction. You would swear it's cancer! Since there is now an effective treatment for FIP, don't discount this as an option. Getting an actual diagnosis could save the cat's life!

1. **Initial diagnostics to rule out systemic causes:**
    a. CBC, Chemistry, electrolytes, T4, urinalysis, Fecal, FIV/Felv snap test (if not on file/ warranted)

2. **Next steps if the above tests come back normal:**
    a. Perform a second fecal +/- fecal PCR
        i. Some parasites shed intermittently, so think of this as your "second check."
        ii. Fecal PCR will pick up on viruses, bacteria and harder to detect organisms

    b. Abdominal ultrasound
        i. You can consider x-rays if you do not have ultrasound capabilities, but they are not as high yield in these cases. They function as a generic health screen and will not pick up on subtle changes. It would be better to have an owner save for an ultrasound if you are at this stage with financial limitations.

    c. Texas GI blood panel
        i. Make sure it includes TLI/PLI/Cobalamin/Folate.
        ii. The cat must be fasted for this test. It is helpful in ruling out EPI, evaluating intestinal function, and raising suspicion of lymphoma.

    d. Gastrointestinal aspirates or biopsies
        i. Can determine together if it is best to do a biopsy via abdominal exploratory vs. fine needle aspirate of a lesion or thickening found on ultrasound. Biopsies will always be superior.

ii. From Dr. Jess: Remember which things are likely to be high yield...
   1. Generally thickened intestines & associated moderate lymphadenopathy: FNA of those lymph nodes won't tell small cell vs. IBD
   2. Specific intestinal masses/really thick ICJ: lymphoma tends to shed more than carcinoma, the top two differentials, so if you get low yield samples you'll get more worried about carcinoma, BUT FIP and feline sclerosing fibroplasia also usually yield low cells too!

STEP 4: Treatment plan:

1. **Diet trial:** Most ideal recommendation is a hypoallergenic diet trial for at least 2 weeks (start the clock when feeding 100% hypo diet). Stool improvement should occur by 1-2 weeks, and the patient's weight should be stabilized. Remember that improvements to your patient's skin will take 6-8 weeks. When performing the diet trial, ensure they are strict and do not get anything additional. You can move through the options based on your patient's response. If the pet is not improving on the current diet by at least 2 weeks, it may be time to try the next listed diet option. Many prescription diets can be refunded if not effective, so prepare to try several options.

   a. Start here: IBD diet trial with Hill's Z/D (dry and wet), Purina HA, or Royal Canin HP. The RC formula does not have a canned version. It only comes in dry but is good for cats that also have urinary issues due to S+Ox index.
      i. Dr. Jess states that there is emerging evidence that cats and dogs may respond better to one hypoallergenic diet over another, so it may take several 2-4 week trials with at least two different hypo diets.

   b. Next options to try: Fiber responsive trial with Hill's W/D, Hill's GI Biome, or Royal Canin GI Fiber Response.
      i. Dr. Jess states that she loves Hill's GI Biome for these cats and dogs with the combo of feeding wet and dry. She also states that for fiber diets, it does not need to be the only diet they eat to be effective. You can use these foods as a base with another food mixed in or on top. This can improve compliance for finicky eaters.

   c. Other final options to try: Reference the chronic vomiting chapter for additional options that may help regarding GI diets or over the counter options.

2. **Fenbendazole trial:** We do a 50 mg/kg dose PO for 5 days.
    a. Example dose for a 10 lb cat (If using liquid at 100 mg/mL): Give 2.3 mL by mouth once a day for 5 days. Repeat in 3 weeks.
        i. It is ok to mix in canned food. Another option is the powder, which is dosed on weight.

3. **Probiotic trial:**
    a. **Proviable:** This is a probiotic used to improve diarrhea. Consider starting a probiotic with the diet change.
        i. The Proviable kit comes with a paste where your owner can give the paste and probiotic capsule simultaneously to improve symptoms.
            1. Give 1 mL of the paste 3x/day for 2-3 days (comes in the Proviable kit).
            2. You will also have them give the capsule daily that they can mix in wet food. It may be best to stay on long term.

    b. **Fortiflora:** This is another probiotic we like to use.
        i. Mix one packet over food once daily. It may be best to stay on long term due to its palatability and ease of administration. It can improve appetite, as many cats like the taste.
        ii. Ashley actually uses Fortiflora to help her cat take her medication. She puts the pill on top of her cat's wet food, and then sprinkles Fortiflora over top. She eats it right up, avoiding pilling.

    c. **Visbiome:** A newer probiotic gaining traction.
        i. **Side note for dogs:** At the 2025 ACVIM Forum, experts released pre-publication guidelines for diagnosing and treating chronic inflammatory enteropathies in dogs. The panel emphasized dietary therapy as the primary treatment and recommended restricting antibiotic use. For probiotics, **Visbiome® Vet (De Simone Formulation)** was the only product to receive a stand-alone recommendation with moderate evidence, while *Saccharomyces boulardii* earned a conditional recommendation when used alongside immunosuppressive therapy. Full guideline publication is expected in January 2026.

4. **Antibiotic Trial:**

    a. Use of metronidazole, amoxicillin, or tylosin has officially fallen out of favor due to concern for dysbiosis, antibiotic resistance, etc. We did start our careers treating diarrhea with this drug, so you will see it mentioned in the first edition. However, we both have shifted away from its routine use for acute diarrhea. You will find many pet owners ask for this drug because of past practices so it is important that you have a good spiel as to why it is no longer recommended to avoid an upset client.

        i. **Example spiel for client requesting metronidazole:**

            1. "I know diarrhea is stressful to see, so I want to explain why we don't automatically use metronidazole anymore for straightforward diarrhea. Recent studies in dogs have shown that metronidazole doesn't help dogs get better faster than doing supportive care alone. It also negatively impacts their healthy bacteria, and most dogs recover within a few days with rest, a digestible diet, fiber and probiotics."

            2. "We're also more cautious with antibiotics now because using them when they aren't truly needed can contribute to antibiotic resistance. Over time, that can make infections harder to treat for both pets and people. So we save antibiotics like metronidazole for situations where they're really necessary and most effective."

        ii. **Dr. Jess shares how she approaches this here**:

            1. Specific instances I would trial antibiotics would be of course if there were signs of active infection (fever, neutrophilia, etc). Sometimes I will look at folate levels and if they are significantly elevated, particularly if things like probiotics and fiber haven't worked, I'll give antibiotics a go, supported with probiotics (beneficial bacterial and yeast is a consideration to give while giving antibiotics as yeast won't be killed off by the antibiotics). Even better if I have a fecal PCR panel because I can at least see if I want to address Clostridium overgrowth or anything like that.

            2. **Side communication tip (especially for dogs with bloody diarrhea):** One now-outdated "rule of thumb" for when to use antibiotics was if there was blood in the stool because of theoretical increased risk for sepsis, but that is not the case unless they have other reasons to worry about immune compromise (geriatric, diabetic, immunosuppressant therapy, etc). We know dogs are much more prone to developing bloody, mucoid stool as part of a gastroenteritis process than people because we see it nearly daily! However to an owner, this is very scary and not

normal. They are probably using humans as a reference point, and it is not normal for a person to have bloody stool, and its presence being a significant cause for concern. So when talking to owners, I find it is really useful to specifically address this difference between dogs and people in terms of severity of disease, prognosis, etc. People are often very relieved when you tell them that dogs have different anatomic responses to colonic inflammation and the blood is neither unusual nor a horribly bad thing on its own (of course still treat it seriously, but this can help a lot with owner compliance!).

iii. Here are some articles if you want to learn more:
   1. https://www.mdpi.com/2813-9372/2/2/19
   2. https://pubmed.ncbi.nlm.nih.gov/39279199/

5. **Other medications to help symptoms in short vs. long term:**

   a. Pectin or probiotic formulated paste (Included in Proviable kit, Vetoquinol Pro-Pectalin oral paste)

   b. Fiber: the prescription diets mentioned above can be utilized (and mixed into the cat's existing food if finicky), Fiber One cereal, or soaked chia seeds into the food (cat's don't mind the taste!)

6. **Vitamin B12 (cyanocobalamin) trial (1000 mcg/ml):**

   a. It is best to have a Texas GI panel performed before this is started to confirm low cobalamin levels. However, if unable, then give it a try. Studies have now shown oral is as effective as the injection, so you can do whichever is easiest for an owner.

   b. For B12 protocols, we recommend using the Texas A&M protocols: https://vetmed.tamu.edu/gilab/research/cobalamin-information/

   c. We usually start seeing improvement after the fourth injection, though you do not want to stop this treatment prematurely.

Dr. Jess Tip

B12 is a water-soluble vitamin so there's no concern for toxicity (they urinate out what they don't need). BUT B12 is a pretty cheap test, so I strongly recommend getting the blood and THEN giving a dose because otherwise you've lost the ability to use it as a diagnostic test. It can be very useful to determine severity of disease, response to treatment, and if considering biopsies, whether the ileum is definitely needed for sampling (where B12 is absorbed).

7. **Steroid trial:**
    a. Prednisolone 1-2 mg/kg/day of lean body weight based on where the tablets fit best.
        i. Remember, if you use this medication without an ultrasound, you may not be able to give them a diagnosis later. Explain to the owner that you are treating with your "best guess," so it could mask the diagnosis if they opt to pursue diagnostics later.
        ii. For most cats (12 lbs+), this amounts to prednisolone 5 mg tablet: 1 tablet PO BID x6 weeks, then go to SID x4 weeks, and then taper to the lowest effective dose. Some cats can maintain well on every other day dosing, while others need a daily low dose.
            1. If the cat is responding well to the medication, Dr. Jess will taper a lot faster at around 2-4 weeks.
        iii. **Note:** Do not forget that cats cannot metabolize prednisone into the active form, so you need to give them prednisolone for best results.
        iv. **Client communication tip:** WARN them about the potential major side effects like diabetes and steroid-induced congestive heart failure. Unfortunately, we have seen both complications occur.

Dr. Jess Tip

With prednisolone dosing, I rarely use more than 2mg/kg per day (2mg/kg BID is WAY too much). And I recommend rounding down, so if deciding between 1.5-2mg/kg/day, I will pick the pill size that is closer to 1.5mg/kg/day to start.

8. **If Prednisone alone does not work:**
    a. Reconsider imaging or biopsy if these have not been done. Next medication to consider is Chlorambucil 2mg per cat PO every 48-72 hours (usually added onto prednisolone dose)
        i. Due to concerns regarding myelosuppression, perform a CBC every 2-3 weeks for the first 3 months of treatment to monitor for trends. Then, you can perform every 6 months for maintenance screening, based on what an owner can afford.
        ii. **Note:** Make sure your client understands that this is a chemotherapy agent so they need to wear gloves when handling and that anyone pregnant/nursing/kids/immunocompromised should not handle this drug.

Here is an example plan that we feel is reasonable approach for many chronic diarrhea cats

1. **Initial exam:**

    a. Prep your owner that there is a long differential list for chronic diarrhea, and your first step is to rule out metabolic disease and obvious parasites **through bloodwork (see initial diagnostic section) and a fecal.** We describe it as an easy first step that is minimally invasive to get a baseline health screen on their cat. If the cat is stable, we will send this lab work out.

        i. Dr. Jess mentions that if an owner is financially able and getting blood on the cat is stressful, add on a B12 +/- fPLi (not SNAP) to look for chronic pancreatitis and malabsorption all at once. It only takes 1-2 months for a cat to become B12 deficient.

    b. **Initiate first treatment plan.** We often get the cat started with **a diet trial, prophylactic course of dewormer (whether we see parasites or not), and a probiotic trial (treatments 1-3 above)** while we wait for lab work results. Explain your first treatment plan, which can address a variety of simple causes with these changes.

        i. Stress that probiotics and a diet change can take 2-4 weeks before improvement or resolution is seen. Different diets may need to be tried as the right one for their cat is found. **Set expectations so that they understand the process** because owners can get frustrated early on.

    c. Set up a **recheck with you in 2-4 weeks.** Diligent follow-up is important so that you can work on the diagnosis and treatment in a methodical way. We often do another one after this at the 6-8 week mark.

        i. Prep them at the recheck visit that you will assess for any improvement, re-evaluate weight, and make a plan for moving forward based on how their cat is doing. **Let the owner know that if the patient is not improving at some point that the next steps are abdominal ultrasound +/- Texas GI panel.** The goal is to figure out the exact cause because treating without diagnostics can mask the disease, making diagnosis more difficult later on. Some owners may have financial concerns preventing more diagnostics at rechecks and that is ok. Focus on getting them back for a recheck so that you can reassess and make adjustments to their treatments based on clinical signs. Never forget to get a weight!

ii. Inform all owners that if their cat is to worsen at any point, recommend they call and let you know right away or come in immediately.

Client communication summary at initial exam of chronic diarrhea cat

- Chronic diarrhea can be frustrating and have many causes.
- You will be working through finding the cause in a step by step manner.
- It is very important that we do rechecks as recommended and follow plans as directed.
- If your first initial plan (diet, probiotics, and dewormer) does not work and if nothing is found on blood work, then the next step will be determined at the recheck in 2-4 weeks with consideration for further diagnostics. You can discuss more then, based on their cat's response.
- Call if the patient worsens at any point.
- Warn about steroid induced CHF and diabetes when prescribing.
- Remember, many prescription diets can be refunded if not effective, so prepare them to try several options. Provide moral support through diet transitions so that they don't give up in the process. Humanize that failing one does not mean there isn't a diet out there that can help and acknowledge the expense/hassle.
    - Dr. Jess shared that there is a bowl that is popular for dogs called Enjoyabowl, and it might work for some cats! www.enjoyabowlaroma.com

2. **First recheck exam at 2-4 weeks:**

    a. After 2-4 weeks of diet, course of dewormer, and probiotic trial, it is time for your recheck to see what may have changed. Check to see if there is **any improvement via history, weight, and your full physical exam.** Touch base on the next diagnostic steps if the owner feels there is no improvement at all. The more you mention next steps, the more on board an owner can be over time. Continue diet, probiotic, and ensure the owner gave the entire course of dewormer.

    b. This is **the point where you can decide if the cat will benefit from treatments 4-6 mentioned above** as well. These additional treatments are considered if the cat's diarrhea is the exact same. Set up a recheck exam for another 3-4 weeks out and certainly sooner if their cat worsens at any time.

3. **Second recheck exam at 6-8 weeks:**

    a. Reassess if there is any improvement via history, weight, and your full physical exam. Ensure compliance. **If not improving, mention next steps of diagnostics** (abdominal ultrasound, biopsies/FNA, Texas GI panel, etc.) **or prednisolone trial (treatment 7)** if they do not wish to pursue advanced testing. Once again, stress the "masking of diagnosis" if they choose to go forward with prednisolone therapy without diagnostics.

Client communication summary at recheck exams for chronic diarrhea cat

- Discuss if any improvement.
- Discuss next steps with diagnostics and treatments.
- Reiterate expectations.
- Urge them to continue diet and probiotics at this point even if there is no improvement.
- Prepare them for next steps should this not work.

NOTES:

NOTES:

NOTES:

Chronic Kidney Disease in Cats

Reviewed by Dr. Jessica Romine, DVM, DACVIM

As a new veterinarian, this is one disease that can really surprise you with how well many patients do with therapy. These patients will present to you with some showing minimal side effects of the disease to others who appear to be presenting on death's doorstep. Owners will also vary on how willing they are to treat, as some will not want their pet to suffer the moment their dehydration becomes clinical, while others will continue treatment to an arguably poor quality of life.

Early detection is key with this disease, as it is a more favorable prognosis when caught early. As you know, you cannot cure it without a kidney transplant. You can only delay progression, so routine screening for early detection and subsequent monitoring is the key to a longer life span with these patients. This will be a major selling point to owners on why it is important to perform wellness blood work annually on younger patients and every six months on senior patients.

Important insight from Dr. Jess:

Young cats basically don't get "early onset CKD." If this is a cat that is young to middle-aged, find the reason because it might be reversible! Ultrasound +/- x-rays for stones (very common cause, especially in Ragdolls and associated breeds), "big kidney little kidney" syndrome, chronic nephritis/infection, polycystic kidney disease, strokes...

Don't forget that if only one kidney is being obstructed by a stone, the other kidney will do the job and you might not detect any changes on bloodwork. Instead, you may see a cat that is acting painful, vomiting, etc. and may get better with supportive care, but if the second one gets hit later on, azotemia appears.

Fun fact: Idexx labs analyzed data from more than a quarter million preventative care profiles of both dogs and cats that were run as wellness blood work to get these amazing statistics. You can use this data to "show the value" of why routine lab work is so important.

Their data, seen below, shows the number of pets that had bloodwork abnormalities indicating follow up was needed.

- **1 in 7 adults**
  - Cats aged 2-8 years
  - Dogs aged 3-6 years
- **1 in 5 seniors**
  - Cats aged 9-13 years
  - Dogs aged 7-10 years
- **2 in 5 geriatrics**
  - Cats aged 14+ years
  - Dogs aged 11+ years

CKD Quick Reference

Signalment: common in senior cats >10 years old. Uncommon in young cats: consider congenital, toxin, stones, etc. See above note from Dr. Jess regarding young cats.

Common clinical signs: weight loss, anorexia, vomiting, nausea, weakness, muscle atrophy, polyuria, polydipsia, stomatitis, oral ulcers, peripheral neuropathies, and seizures

Diagnosis:

- Azotemia (elevation of BUN and creatinine). Check IRIS staging for diagnosis. Warning: some pets have azotemia even though their levels are still 'normal' on the lab reference range. Pay attention to the actual values for diagnosis, not whether it is in the 'red' or not!
- Isosthenuria (USG 1.008-1.012; cats can often be up to 1.020)
- Elevation of SDMA (raises suspicion and is a sensitive, early marker). If seen without azotemia, see Idexx algorithm.
- Elevated UPC

Other abnormalities you should look for if CKD is suspected:

- Hypertension
- Heart disease
- Urinary tract infection
- Pyelonephritis
- Anemia
- Ulceration (oral, GI, other)/Melena
- Stones or mineralizations of kidneys

Treatment:

- **Asymptomatic and IRIS Stage 1:** Change to a kidney specific diet. We love Purina NF early care or Hill's K/D Early Care at this stage. However, please note that there is growing evidence not to overly restrict protein in early stages. Our key takeaway? It isn't the end of the world if the cat won't eat a kidney diet yet or the client is not ready to commit. Encourage and recommend feeding wet food to focus on hydration. Purina Hydracare is another great product to consider!
- **Mild to moderately symptomatic and IRIS Stage 2-3:** Adjust diet to Hill's K/D, Purina NF advanced care, or RC Renal Support Formulas. Continue focus on hydration through wet food and consider Purina Hydracare. Script out medications to manage symptoms like appetite stimulants, anti-emetics, etc.
- **Moderate to severely symptomatic and IRIS stage 3-4:** More aggressive therapy may need to be started, such as hospitalization for fluid therapy, daily subcutaneous fluids, but will ultimately be based on the stability of your patient.

What is an SDMA test?: This is a newer test that many laboratories add on to wellness blood work panels, and it is short for symmetric dimethylarginine. It is a serum test and indicates a declining glomerular filtration rate in dogs and cats. This value increases as kidney function decreases, regardless of the underlying cause. It will elevate due to acute, active, or chronic injury.

- Idexx has a great algorithm on their website you can refer to if you find an elevation in SDMA without an elevation of BUN or creatinine. Do not forget that if you are ever in doubt, call Idexx or Antech for a free consultation with one of their internal medicine specialists. This is an invaluable, free resource to help you determine appropriate treatments for patients.

- **Tip from Dr. Jess:** If you get a normal SDMA and high creatinine, trust the creatinine. Other diseases, especially cachexic GI diseases, can also raise SDMA.

- Urinalysis will always be an important next step to gain valuable information in the face of an elevation in SDMA.

So, you have diagnosed a cat with kidney disease. Now, what?

1. Determine what **IRIS stage** your patient is in.

    a. Staging allows you to determine the best treatment and monitoring plan for your patient moving forward. You will adjust therapies over time, as your patient progresses through the stages. Refer to this website for detail on staging based on creatinine, SDMA, blood pressure, and UPC:

    https://www.idexx.com/files/Stagingpdf.pdf

    b. Obtain a urinalysis and a blood pressure if not done yet (Reference case one below for blood pressure tips.). This will help with staging but also explain to owners, that many cats have undiagnosed hypertension and UTIs. Not every owner will pursue this, but it should be mentioned since hypertension can cause other health concerns such as blindness, strokes, etc. and UTIs can progress to severe renal insult with cats. Routine checking of these parameters is especially important for cats that are symptomatic for kidney disease or have sudden behavior changes (which can often be attributed to hypertension). Be sure to mention the clinical signs noted in the chart above so that they can monitor for signs of disease progression at home.

2. Determine your **treatment plan** based on their stage.

    a. The **two goals of treatment** are to **delay progression** of the disease by preserving remaining kidney function and to **reduce symptoms** in order to improve patient comfort.

    b. Refer to these websites we like to reference for details on treatment based on age:
        i. https://www.idexx.com/files/Treatmentpdf.pdf
        ii. http://www.iris-kidney.com/pdf/IRIS_CAT_Treatment_Recommendations_2019.pdf
        iii. https://static1.squarespace.com/static/666b9ec-b4064a156963b4162/t/66a6dc1dbfaa20426da8e99b/1722211357641/IRIS_CAT_Treatment_Recommendations_2023.pdf

Above is a brief overview of kidney disease to refresh your memory and give you some quick resources we like to use in general practice. Vet school taught you how to diagnose and treat chronic kidney disease, so now it is time for the good stuff. It is time to practice your client communication when managing this disease because believe us when we say that you will have a HUGE range of client interactions here. There will be some clients who have been through this before with another cat and do not want their cat to suffer, while there are others who will want to hospitalize their cat every single time they become symptomatic. Some of your cat patients will look like they will not live another forty-eight hours, but then they will bounce back and live another six months. Cats can be such troopers with this disease, so there are some important points you will want to communicate to owners to make sure you are always on the same page.

Common components of an at home treatment plan

Depending on which stage your CKD patient is in, these treatments can give many cats a good quality of life. The goal is to delay progression with diet and manage symptoms so that the cat has less GI upset, adequate hydration, and a better appetite. **You can start with 1-2 components, and then build over time as the disease progresses.**

Here is an example of our at home treatment plan for clients that will include one or several of the following components:

- **Diet:** Diet is the mainstay of chronic kidney disease management, as it is the ONLY thing proven to slow its progression. Nearly every cat will be on this diet (though towards the end stages, we find some develop an aversion to them). Diets include Hill's K/D, Purina NF, and Royal Canin Renal Support. All three companies have an early care version as well that is specially formulated for cats based on the stage they are in. The early care/ support versions of kidney diets aim to keep a cat's weight and muscle mass stable for as long as possible.

Dr. Jess Tip

Encourage wet food if you can! Hydracare is also good to trial now, and experimenting with preferred water methods (fountain, porcelain, wide & flat, glass, raised slightly if they're arthritic, etc)

  - **Diet options:** Your first choice is for the owner to feed a canned renal diet, if they will eat it (any of the flavors!). Second choice is a dry renal diet. Last choice is any wet food so that they can maintain hydration. If they refuse all of these options, have your owner offer anything they will eat. The truth is that cats ultimately determine their own treatment to a certain regard. We do the best we can here with offering options, as we know diet can have a big impact on disease progression. However, in the end stages, our highest priority is for the cat to eat. The balanceit.com website can be considered if the owner is open to a home cooked option.

  - **Food intolerances in cats:** Cats develop food intolerances EASILY with CKD. They are often nauseous, and cats are notorious for linking their diets to nausea. This is why we do not like to feed these diets to them when they are sick and hospitalized. It can cause them to develop resistance to their diets so try to avoid it.
    - An option that can be considered in hospital for an inappetent cat (despite PO appetite stimulants) or for at home management if you have an owner that is comfortable with its management is placement of an esophageal tube. They can feed slurried kidney diets through it or the Royal Canin renal liquid diet. E-tubes are often underutilized and can be a great way for a client to medicate, hydrate and feed a cat that may need some extra TLC to get through a transition period of this disease.

- **Supportive medications:** In the early stages of renal disease, cats often do not need these yet. Once clinical signs develop, we use whichever combination below feels most appropriate for the cat. Remember to prioritize and keep it simple because we all know medicating cats can be difficult.
  - **A medication update from our first edition:** At this time, there is no good evidence that giving stomach-protecting medications preventively helps dogs or cats with early to moderate kidney disease (IRIS stages 1-3). For pets with more advanced kidney disease (IRIS stage 4), we still don't have clear answers, and more research is needed to know whether these medications are truly beneficial.
    - Source: Marks, S. L., Kook, P. H., Papich, M. G., Tolbert, M. K., & Willard, M. D. (2018). ACVIM consensus statement: Support for rational administration of gastrointestinal protectants to dogs and cats. Journal of Veterinary Internal Medicine, 32(6), 1823–1840. https://doi.org/10.1111/jvim.15337

Further information on use of PPIs in our patients

Omeprazole was not considered helpful in these conditions unless there was clear evidence of stomach ulcers or inflammation of the esophagus.

- Renal disease (acute kidney injury (AKI) or CKD IRIS stage 1, 2, or 3)
- Pancreatitis
- GI foreign body
- Dietary indiscretion
- GI surgery
- Inflammatory bowel disease
- Low grade intestinal lymphoma
- Non-specific GI signs of inappetence, vomiting, weight loss, diarrhea of unknown etiology
- Hepatic disease with no evidence of concurrent portal hypertension.

Sainz Á, García-Sancho M, Villaescusa A, Rodríguez-Franco F, Díaz-Regañón D, Olmeda P, Marks SL. Prevalence and appropriateness of omeprazole prescription in dogs at a veterinary teaching hospital before and after the publication of the ACVIM consensus statement on the rational administration of gastrointestinal protectants. Front Vet Sci.2024;11:1352496. doi:10.3389/fvets.2024.1352496

- **Antiemetic:**
    - **Cerenia/maropitant** (16 mg: Give ¼ tablet PO q24-48 hrs): Check this dosage to make sure it works for your cat, as this is a common chronic dosing regimen for the vast majority of our patients. You can safely use this medication chronically in cats. Cerenia tablets are used off label at this time. Only Cerenia injection is on label at the time of our publishing.

- **Appetite stimulant:**
    - **Mirataz Transdermal** (1.5 inch strip applied gently to the inside of the ear once daily; rotate ears each day): This is the easiest to administer. The owner must wear gloves when administering to the inside of the cat's ear. See packet instructions for full details, as it guides the owner through precise administration.
        - Side note: Transdermal medications must be discontinued or decreased to every 3-5 days if the ear is becoming very red and/or hot to the touch. This is a common side effect of this formulation. Oftentimes, it is due to the owner rubbing in the medication too much. The company describes its administration to be "similar to icing a cake," so that is a good way to describe it to owners.
        - There is a caution about its use in cats with kidney and hepatic disease. However, we have both safely used it in these patients.
    - **Mirtazapine tablets** (1.8 mg/cat q24-48 hr OR 3.75 mg/cat PO q72 hrs)
    - **Elura** (capromorelin oral solution- 2 mg/kg PO q24 hr): Cats don't often love the vanilla taste, so owners will often see excessive drooling with its use. It helps to warn them of this but tends to work well!

- **Subcutaneous fluids:** We often do not add this treatment in until later stages of renal disease. Owners can bring the pet into the clinic for administration several times a week or administer at home if they feel comfortable doing so. If the owner is administering at home, be sure to tell them to contact you if they feel this treatment is creating added stress for their cat. Some cats start avoiding owners if it is performed too frequently, and in those situations owners often feel that the bond they have with their cat is becoming strained. This would be a reason to decrease or suspend its use.

- **Maintenance fluids are often used such as Normosol R, Plasmalyte, LRS, etc.**
  - Common doses used are between 50-150 mL/cat several times a week depending on the size of the cat and heart status. We often start with twice a week or every other day based on the severity of the patient.
    - **Tip from Dr. Jess:** Have clients monitor baseline respiratory rates while sleeping (RR <30) to help them identify potential fluid overload as fluid doses progress over time

- For those administering fluids at home, you want to teach them how to do this in person. This is something a technician can teach a client during the first administration. This website can be a valuable reference for them too.
  - https://icatcare.org/advice/how-to-give-subcutaneous-fluids-to-your-cat/

- **Other miscellaneous medications:** Some other medications we consider as blood work abnormalities develop are...

  - Purina Hydracare
  - Phosphorus binders (Epakitin powder is an example product.)
  - Potassium supplementation (Renal K gel is an example product.)
  - Calcitriol
  - Vitamin B12 injections
  - Drugs to treat anemia:
    - Darbepoetin (injectable): drug used from human medicine
    - Varenzin (molidustat oral suspension): preferred alternative to Darbopoetin that is now available
      - **Insight from Dr. Jess:** This drug is an oral feline-specific EPO stimulator without the significant risks of antibodies developing, and it can be started sooner with more efficacy. I usually find it takes at least 2 rounds (bottles) to see the PCV going up!

Three CKD case examples with treatment plans and client communication points

Now, we are going to talk you through three real life examples of how CKD can look out in practice. We will discuss how to best present your plan to clients, key communication points, and actual treatment plans based on these cases.

CKD CASE 1: **Azotemia found on routine blood work of an older cat.**

You have a 12 year FS DSH who is presenting for her annual exam. The owner has no concerns, and they feel like she is doing very well. On exam, you notice that she has lost 1.5 pounds from her previous visit six months ago. She is 10% overweight with mild dental disease, but you notice no other abnormalities. You recommend annual blood work and use the handy dandy data above to convince the owner that it is worth doing today, especially considering her cat's unexpected weight loss. You get your results back and find a mildly elevated BUN, normal creatinine, elevated SDMA, and isosthenuria (1.015).

You have just diagnosed your first case of early kidney disease in an asymptomatic patient. What do you say to your owner?

Our go-to way to communicate to difficult news to clients:

Connection → Information → Reassurance → Next Steps
This flow helps provide clarity, emotional support and ensures client understanding.

- **Veterinarian:** *"Hi Mrs. Jones, I hope you're doing well today. I just got back Panda's blood work results. Is now a good time to go over them together?" (Wait for confirmation)*
- **Veterinarian:** *"Ok great. So, the majority of Panda's blood work looks good. However, there were a few changes on her chemistry panel and urinalysis that I'd like to talk through with you."*
- **Veterinarian:** *"Specifically, we're seeing some early signs of kidney disease. Her kidney values are mildly elevated, and her urine is more dilute than it should be, which tells us her kidneys aren't filtering quite as well as they should."*

- **Veterinarian:** *"The good news is that Panda isn't showing many outward symptoms right now, aside from weight loss. And that gives us an opportunity to step in early. While we can't reverse kidney disease, we can slow it down and help her feel as good as possible for as long as possible."*
- **Veterinarian:** *"Based on the results, it looks like Panda has less than 25% kidney function remaining. That may sound concerning, but many cats can still live comfortably, often for one to three years or more with the right support and monitoring."*
- **Veterinarian:** *"Do you have any questions so far before we talk about what the next steps would look like?"* (Wait for questions, respond with empathy and clarity.)
- **Veterinarian:** *"Let's go ahead and talk through what we'll do next. We'll want to run a few additional tests to better understand what stage of kidney disease Panda is in, and based on that, we can adjust her treatment plan at home to better support her kidneys moving forward."*

Next steps with your patient:

1. **Recommend the client schedule a follow-up appointment for further diagnostics.** This will help rule out any further pre-renal or post-renal causes as well as help determine the cat's exact IRIS stage.

    a. **Baseline blood pressure screen:** Try to do it in the bottom of the cat carrier or in the clients lap where the cat appears most comfortable.

        i. Before starting blood pressure medications, make sure the cat was calm during the readings. If you have any doubt, consider asking the owner to do a follow-up blood pressure check in a week with the cat where the cat is given a low dose of gabapentin at home two hours prior to the visit. Owners are usually ok with this understanding the importance of controlling blood pressure and also the caution we want to take before starting their pet on a potentially lifelong medication.

        ii. If hypertension is present, start your patient on either amlodipine (current starting dose recommendations are 0.625 mg/cat PO q24 hrs) or telmisartan (new liquid FDA approved medication called Semintra).

iii. When starting a blood pressure medication, recheck blood pressure at an appropriate time interval (usually within 1-2 weeks of starting the medication) and have owners monitor for any signs of low blood pressure like weakness and collapse.

b. **UPC:** This test helps with IRIS staging. A UPC can also be helpful to be sure you are managing both the kidney disease and hypertension appropriately with the medication. If one or both are still elevated, medications like benazepril can be added in at this point.
   i. Though UPC testing is not routinely done, it is a part of the staging process and helps you determine if further medications are indicated. Significant proteinuria on your urinalysis is a good clue that this test is of higher priority. However, in cost conscious owners, it may not be routinely performed.

c. **+/- Imaging** (x-rays, ultrasound): This will help look at the size/shape of kidneys, other organs and allow you to go on a stone hunt. You may find results that can be treated, monitored or that can lend into prognosis (signs of cancer, surgery or dissolution diet to remove stones, etc.).

2. **When do you start a kidney diet and how do you communicate about it?:** This is the mainstay of treatment at IRIS stage 2 to help delay progression of renal disease. Research shows that starting a kidney diet when in IRIS stage 2 can improve life expectancy for up to two years. Many cats will live longer than that too!

   a. Client communication tips around kidney diets:
      i. Explain to the owner what the diet is doing so that they understand the science behind the cost. Some nutritional highlights we mention are reduced phosphorus and protein to decrease the workload of the kidney, decrease toxins, and other added antioxidants are present for kidney health like omega 3 fatty acids.
      ii. Make sure the client understands that this should be the ONLY thing their cat eats, as other foods will provide the protein and phosphorus the prescription diets are trying to minimize. Let them know there are various types out there so if their cat does not like one, you can prescribe another. Each company has sample kits you can sell to clients to have their cat taste them to see which ones they like best. Pet food companies will also reimburse a client if they

purchase a food and their cat will not eat it. These are good selling points, since many owners feel cats are picky.

iii. Explain that in later stages of the disease, some cats may not like the diets or stop eating the diet as the disease progresses. Be sure the client lets you know if that happens, as we may have other prescription options that have not been tried, or you can recommend they try a good quality wet food to help with hydration. Their cat maintaining its weight and health are most important in the later stages.

3. **Set expectations and follow-up plan:** Mrs. Jones set up a follow up visit and opted to do a blood pressure (came back normal) and abdominal/thoracic films (came back normal). You have staged her cat as an IRIS stage 1.

- **Veterinarian:** *"Mrs. Jones, now that we've completed all the necessary tests and have a clearer picture of Panda's condition at stage 1, I'd like to talk about the next steps in managing her kidney disease."*
- *"While this condition will worsen over time, our main goals moving forward are to maintain her weight and keep her well-hydrated. Both of which are really important in slowing the progression and keeping her comfortable."*
- *"If possible, I recommend feeding her a* ***wet food-only diet****, as canned food naturally contains more moisture, which supports kidney function. It also tends to be more palatable and can help with weight maintenance. Any diet she loves is fine, but aiming for wet food is key. Eventually, we will discuss a kidney specific diet when her kidney stage changes."*
- *"Make sure Panda has* ***access to fresh water throughout the house:*** *some cats drink more if there are multiple bowls around the house or if you use a* ***cat water fountain,*** *which many cats prefer. Another option to consider is* ***Purina Hydra Care,*** *which is a hydration supplement designed specifically for cats and can help support fluid intake even more."*
- *"My recommendation is to have Panda come in every six months for an exam, blood work, and blood pressure. This helps us monitor for any new concerns like low potassium, rising phosphorus, increased kidney values, GI issues, or weight loss. If anything concerning comes up between visits, like changes in appetite, vomiting, or increased thirst or urination, please reach out sooner."*
- *"As the disease progresses, we may need to add more treatments to keep her comfortable like anti-nausea medications or appetite stimulants. We'll take it one step at a time and adjust her care based on how she's doing."*

Client communication summary for azotemia found on routine blood work

- CKD is irreversible, and it will progress.
- Many cats can do well with this disease, and it is important to work together as a team.
- We can slow its progression down by improving and maintaining hydration as well as a kidney specific diet when appropriate.
- Long term monitoring of blood work, urinalysis, and blood pressure are recommended for these cats. Senior visits every 6 months are ideal to keep up with any changes and adjust therapy as needed.
- With this disease, we add in therapies over time to support them as the disease progresses, which is why close monitoring of blood work and symptoms at home is really important. Examples include anti-nausea medications, appetite stimulants, subcutaneous fluids, etc. An easy example is how some CKD cats start eating less bc of excess gastric acid, which can be helped with omeprazole,etc.
- Go over symptoms of kidney disease or hypertension for owners to look out for at home.

CKD CASE 2: **Severely azotemic 15 yr old cat with a heart murmur.**

You have a walk-in emergency that is a 15 year old MN DLH. He has never been seen at your hospital before, and the owner did not bring medical records with them. He presents with acute vomiting for about three days, hyporexia for the last week, and is lethargic. On exam, you can tell that he is at least 7-8% dehydrated, 20% underweight, has moderate dental disease, has a grade II/VI left parasternal heart murmur, and an unthrifty coat.

- **What questions should you ask the owner?**
  - What is his health history?
  - Any prior diseases I need to know about?
  - Has someone heard a heart murmur on him before?
  - Is it possible he got into anything? (Think toxic plants, ethylene glycol, etc.)
  - Has his diet changed recently?
  - When he vomits, what does it look like?
  - How are his thirst and urination habits?

- Now that you have your history...**What do you want to do next?**

    - High priority in this cat is screening lab work: **CBC, chemistry, T4, urinalysis.**
    - If an owner has available finances, abdominal and thoracic x-rays and a proBNP will be helpful to complete the picture, especially with his heart murmur.

- Results came back with moderate anemia (23%), severe azotemia (BUN-too high to read, needs to be diluted, and a creatinine of 11), hyperphosphatemia (11.9), and a moderate bacterial (rod) urinary tract infection. **If the owner is able to financially, you should now send his urine off for culture to ensure you treat the infection appropriately.** These cats are at risk for pyelonephritis.

Treatment options: Now what?? You have three options for this cat: hospitalization (best option to try to get this cat stabilized and feeling better), outpatient therapy (an option, but not recommended), or humane euthanasia.

1. **Hospitalization:** This cat is a prime candidate for hospitalization. He is clinically ill and severely dehydrated. He needs intravenous fluids to improve his azotemia, medications to improve nausea/appetite (appetite stimulants, antiemetics), and intravenous antibiotics to treat his urinary tract infection efficiently since he is not eating well. Repeat lab work over his stay will ensure no other complications develop such as hypokalemia, and you will be able to assess his response to therapy.

    a. If your hospital does not hospitalize patients, referral is indicated. This is the best option, as he will benefit from 24 hour monitoring.

    b. If your owner is cost conscious, you can offer to hospitalize at your hospital. Mention to the owner that their cat will still need multiple days of therapy, so they can either drop their cat off each day for treatments while you are open or stay overnight unsupervised. You MUST stress to the owner that no one is watching him overnight, and pets can become disconnected from fluids, chew out catheters, progress clinically, and ultimately no one is there to intervene if something severe happens.

    c. Sample in hospital treatment protocol:
        i. Fluid therapy
            1. **Tip from Dr. Jess:** A cautious bolus to start is appropriate here. Start high then taper, as this will help you see a better response for this patient. If

you just do 2x maintenance, that's probably actually just maintenance for a cat with CKD (who is polyuric, based on isosthenuria!). I usually will do maintenance + rehydration correction (aim for 5-10%; there's no way an anorexic vomiting cat with CKD isn't at least 7% dehydrated!) over 12- 24 hours then taper down. With a cat with a heart murmur, remember that the kidneys are what are life threatening right now and not the potential heart issue. Consider a Pro-BNP to assess the heart, but remember that dehydration & anemia could be causing murmur too.

a. Ways to monitor fluid therapy in a cat with a heart murmur?
    i. RR/RE q2 hour to assess for trends
    ii. tPOCUS q6-8 hour

ii. TPR checks at appropriate intervals
    1. Typically, we perform them q6-8 hr based on abnormalities noted and stress level of the patient.

iii. Cerenia/maropitant
    1. 1 mg/kg IV q24 hr
    2. +/- ondansetron as well, they can be synergistic
    3. Metoclopramide has no anti-nausea properties in cats

iv. Appropriate antibiotics, if a UTI or pyelonephritis is present. *For an ill cat like this one, we would send out a urine culture so we can tailor antibiotics appropriately.*
    1. We often start with ampicillin sulbactam 22 mg/kg IV q8 hr. (Note: When given IV it should be given slowly over 10-15 min.)
    2. If concern for pyelonephritis exists, add in a fluoroquinolone since #1 doesn't penetrate the kidneys well. We tend to give oral here due to potential side effects of IV enrofloxacin (blindness). Our go to is pradofloxacin.

v. +/- Blood pressure medications if warranted

vi. +/- Appetite stimulant

vii. +/- Phosphate binder if eating in hospital

d. Key communication points with this plan:
    i. **Expect 24-72 hours of hospitalization to see how he responds:** We always tell owners the key is to assess his response to therapy over 24-72 hours. If his values are not improving or he worsens despite treatment, then he most likely will not get better. If he improves steadily over 72 hours, he may then

do well with medical management for an extended period of time at home. We like to see these cats start to eat prior to discharge.

1. **Risks of fluids with suspected underlying heart disease:** Warn owners that with treatment in a cat with a heart murmur, we have to be very careful that we do not cause an already bad heart to go into heart failure and that it is something you will be watching closely during hospitalization.
2. **Long term goal:** In these very sick cats, warn owners that unfortunately we could be looking at only weeks to months despite aggressive treatment. We could get lucky and get much longer, but how the cat responds over time will guide us the best.

2. **Aggressive outpatient care:** This is an option, but one we would dissuade owners from choosing due to concern for poor prognosis. The reason is that given the state of this pet, there is concern for poor prognosis and more suffering due to the cat's current clinical signs. We say something like this...

   a. *"We are concerned that this option will be ineffective and prolong him feeling poorly. Given his current state and level of dehydration and infection, I feel he truly needs hospitalization if he is to have a chance to recover. My fear with this option is that it may just prolong his suffering being that he feels pretty lousy right now, and I know you don't want that for him, so I am advising against it."*

   b. This option entails daily subcutaneous fluids, Cerenia, appetite stimulants, oral antibiotics, phosphorus binder (when eating well), and kidney diet. If no improvement within 72 hours or if the cat worsens at any point, humane euthanasia is indicated.

3. **Humane euthanasia:** Though there is a chance for recovery, this option should also be offered to an owner and is reasonable should they choose to pick it.

Client communication: After communicating these three options to the owner, you will want to consider these additional client communication points.

- **Prognosis:** This is a difficult one. The truth is that we do not know how this cat will respond in this case, but we think it is reasonable to try treatment. He may respond well, but he also may not, so you must communicate that to the owner. After discussing the three options with the owner (hospitalization, outpatient care, or humane euthanasia), we ask them if they have any questions. You can reiterate again that if their cat is going to recover from this, aggressive hospitalization will be needed to get him feeling better faster.

- **Reiterate the end goal:** Explain to the owner that the goal is to ensure their cat has a good quality of life. If he is stressed out with our treatments or not responding well, the owner needs to use this response to guide if we need to adjust our plan or if euthanasia is best for their pet. We explain it like this...
    - *"If your cat is not responding to our treatments or goes home and has more bad days than good days, and he is stressed out with our treatments, we need to decide what is best for him. Sometimes, it is better to let our pet go before they are really truly suffering. You have done everything you can for him up to this point. I am here to guide you through this difficult time. What questions do you have for me?"*
    - If you feel like an owner may be "holding on too long," ask what their goals are for their cat. Sometimes, you have to get them to explain their thinking in order to guide them toward the best answer. Directing them to a company like Lap of Love or sharing their resources with them can be helpful so they can talk to them about hospice care, have an objective QOL scale to use, etc.
        - We love: https://www.lapoflove.com/how-will-i-know-it-is-time/lap-of-love-quality-of-life-scale.pdf

- **Follow up plan:** Should the cat do well, recheck blood work 10-14 days after fluid therapy and initial presentation to see how the azotemia is responding, and if improved, kidney diets and subcutaneous fluids tend to give them a good quality of life. You can recommend SQ fluids as often as daily, but we often recommend every 2-3 days initially for patient comfort if the cat feels better clinically. **We have often been surprised here where cats that present "on death's doorstep" turn around and live another 6-12 months.**

Client communication summary for a geriatric, symptomatic cat with CKD and a heart murmur

- Go over findings with your client. Their cat has kidney failure and is VERY sick, causing you to be very concerned for their short term prognosis.
- Go over treatment options. There are three options for treatment: hospitalization, outpatient care, and euthanasia. There are pros and cons to each. Given how sick their cat is, hospitalization is strongly recommended. Outpatient therapy is not a good option and one you fear may lead to prolonged suffering.
- Set a goal to align the owner with your plan. The end goal with therapy is to get their cat back to a good quality of life.
- Caution owner of risks. There is a risk of heart failure when you treat CKD patients that have a pre-existing heart murmur with fluids, so you will be tailoring the fluids closely during your treatment. It is important an owner knows these two diseases are "not best friends."
- Discuss prognosis and expectations. Prognosis varies, and you will need 24-72 hours to see. If the cat worsens over that time, then we will have to consider human euthanasia. If the cat improves, it is important to recheck the cat in 10-14 days to reassess and make a long term plan.

CKD CASE 3: **Patient with pre-existing kidney disease that develops clinical signs.**

Panda, from scenario one, presents to you six months later with acute vomiting, polyuria, polydipsia, inappropriate urination, and 24 hours of anorexia.

What do you recommend?

- Repeat blood work! Let's see what may be going on with her kidneys now that some time has passed. You should perform a **CBC, chemistry, T4, and urinalysis.** Consider checking blood pressure if possible too.

Results came back with a moderate azotemia (BUN is 65 and creatinine is 3.8) and a severe bacterial (cocci) urinary tract infection. Blood pressure is normal. **Again, if the owner is**

financially able too, send her urine off for culture to ensure you treat the infection appropriately. (Ex: Always ask if they can send off culture, but if needed choose treatment over culture when financial limitations.)

Great, now what!?

- **Explain your findings:** Ok, so first things first. You need to explain to your owner what you have found. Panda is now clinical for her kidney disease. It is time to step it up a notch from her original treatment plan of a prescription kidney diet.

- **Offer treatment options (hospitalization vs. outpatient treatment)**

  - **Hospitalization:** It is never wrong to offer hospitalization when a patient is symptomatic. She will certainly improve faster with intravenous fluids and antibiotics. Gung-ho owners will do it.

  - **Outpatient treatment:** Not every owner can afford hospitalization each time their cat becomes ill from kidney disease. If an owner is hesitant to treat or financially restricted, the cat may be a good candidate for outpatient care too. You can always start outpatient care and mention hospitalization as a next step if the cat is not improving or worsening in 24-48 hours.
    - **Example outpatient treatment plan:**
      - **Daily subcutaneous fluids** (It is usually between 10-20 mL/kg: ends up being between 50-150 mL per day based on the size of the cat.) Adjust dose and frequency based on heart status.
      - **Anti-nausea injection** while in hospital (Maropitant subcutaneously is a good choice), then send home with the oral version for long term use as needed.
      - **Phosphate binder:** Dr. Jess loves the aluminum hydroxide powder product from Thriving Pets that is non-flavored and can be added to food easily.
      - **Send home medications:** The goal here is to set the patient up for success but not overwhelm the owner with so many medications that they cannot get into the pet. Giving the owner an order of importance for medications can be very helpful. Alternatively, offer once a day tech appointments for treatments if they are overwhelmed.

- **Antibiotics:** Amoxicillin-clavulanic acid (Clavamox) is the ideal choice. It tends to treat many of these infections. However, if your patient is not eating, this may make the cat more ill with GI side effects. Send out a culture and sensitivity because it will tell you how effective your antibiotic choice is at treating the infection within 3-5 days.
    - Dr. Jess notes on antibiotic choices for this case: Fluoroquinolones are appropriate here, although of course be a judicious antibiotic steward - don't give our more advanced antibiotics unless there's a significant chance of it actually being pyelonephritis. Convenia is NOT as ideal in this case as it has poor kidney penetration and may contribute to resistance. (While the authors have used Convenia for UTIs in select cases (with follow-up cultures to confirm resolution) the presence of azotemia here makes kidney involvement more likely, so an alternative antibiotic is a better choice)
- **Appetite stimulant daily**
- **+/- Cerenia tablets daily**

- **Set up expectations:** Always set up your next follow-up, so the owner knows when to come back in. **If your patient responds well to outpatient care, recheck them in 10-14 days** for a repeat urinalysis, chemistry, and blood pressure. You can ensure the urinary tract infection is resolved and azotemia is improving. If other abnormalities are noted, such as hypokalemia or hyperphosphatemia, you can add in additional therapies at that time.

    - Example: Hyperphosphatemia can be treated with aluminum hydroxide. See IRIS treatment guidelines on when. Be sure to tell the owner:
        - *"If your cat worsens at any point, or the plan is overwhelming, please call us and come back sooner."*

- **Set up a nurse callback for 2-3 days in:** Have a nurse give the owner a call in 2-3 days to make sure the owner and pet are doing ok and to see if they are having any issues with medications. You may give her an 'order of importance' with regards to the cat's medication regimen.

Client communication summary when a patient with pre-existing CKD becomes clinical

- Go over findings. *"Panda's kidney disease has worsened both with symptoms she is showing at home and in blood work. CKD has also caused her to get a secondary UTI."*
- Go over treatment options. *"Her kidney values have jumped high enough this time that hospitalization should be considered. There are two reasonable options: hospitalization or outpatient therapy."* Describe pros and cons of each and cost.
- Set a goal to align the client with a mutual goal. *"The goal is to get her feeling better and to get values back down to a more manageable place where she feels better."*
- Caution owner about back up plan if no improvement.
- Set expectation for course of action if the cat does improve, which is a recheck with you in 10-14 days where you recheck values and discuss components of long term plan at home (ie: daily omeprazole, cerenia tablets prn if needed, biweekly fluids, etc.).

Lastly, there will be many more scenarios that come your way. However, the gist will be the same!

1. Determine the stage of kidney disease your patient is in and how symptomatic the cat is at the time.

2. This will guide your prognosis, treatment recommendations, and follow-up plan.

3. Have a frank conversation with the owner, so you are on the same page from the start. This will guide how much to recommend based on their goals for their cat. You can always readjust your plan if the owner's goals change over time.

    - **Tip from Dr. Jess:** Explain progression of CKD over time because cats rarely have a steady decline but tend to have a sudden drop (infection, other GI upset that dehydrates them, etc.), which if we can stabilize and support, they will then plateau at their new normal with good quality of life for another period of time before another drop. Goals are to draw these plateaus out as long as possible.

For when you need to use a fluoroquinolone:

Dr. Jess Tip: The blindness appears to be enrofloxacin-specific for the large part, and only at higher doses. Here in NZ we only have enrofloxacin, and we standard use 5 mg/kg for cats and 10 mg/kg for dogs.

NOTES:

NOTES:

NOTES:

Chronic Vomiting in Older Cats

Reviewed by Dr. Jessica Romine, DVM, DACVIM

Chronic vomiting will be a very common presenting complaint you see in your older cat patients. These patients come in different presentations. For some, they present acutely ill with rapid weight loss while others may pop up at a yearly appointment where the owner casually mentions their cat vomits 3-4+ times per month. Cats end up having many unique factors surrounding their gastrointestinal tract that make them prone to vomiting. Your differential list is long, and sometimes you will be faced with an owner who is unwilling to perform all the diagnostics you recommend. These cases can seem daunting and make you feel like you do not even know where to start. Don't worry. Here is our basic approach including some empirical treatments that work for us, and a few case examples.

Here is our basic approach:

1. Differentiate vomiting from regurgitation?
2. Confirm acute or chronic vomiting is present
3. If chronic, determine if it is pathologic or 'normal'?
4. Is the underlying cause due to systemic or gastrointestinal disease?
5. Diagnostic plan
6. Treatment plan

STEP 1: Differentiate vomiting from regurgitation?

- Owners do not often know the difference between these two, so ask your questions about if abdominal contractions are present, etc. that guide this differentiation.
  - Tip from Dr. Jess: Timing can also help, and here are some further questions that can help distinguish vomiting from regurgitation.
    - "How soon is the action after eating?"
    - "Is there bile or just foam and undigested kibble?"
    - "Can you hear them "wind up" first or does it just come out?"

- Vomiting is active vs. regurgitation is passive.

STEP 2: Confirm acute or chronic vomiting is present.

- Note: **Acute vomiting** in a sick, young cat could raise higher concern of an obstructive process, especially if no prior history of vomiting.

  - Perform a thorough history asking about any toxin ingestion (such as plants, medications, etc.), recent sewing, playing with string, chewed up toys, etc.
    - Tip from Dr. Jess: Consider if appetite is down too or is it just vomiting present. Are the symptoms more noticeable, frequent, or of larger volume? Is it both water and food coming up?

- Again, history will guide you. Chronic vomiting typically lasts three weeks or more.

STEP 3: If chronic, determine if it is pathologic or normal?

- Few examples:

  - Occasional vomiting in an otherwise healthy cat (a few times per year or every other month that pertains to a hairball) can be normal.
    - Tip from Dr. Jess: Especially in cats that haven't historically had hairballs, starting to bring them up isn't normal to suddenly do and can indicate dysmotility is developing (IBD or otherwise). In long-haired cats, even if they didn't eat a foreign body, hairballs can be a big issue and be obstructive, so don't rule it out even if they're not "the type to eat things!"

- Some healthy cats will eat too quickly and vomit up food right after ingestion. It will typically be whole kibble in the vomit. This can be normal due to fast ingestion, and slower feeding resolves the issue. Ways to help this behavior at home are slow feeders, automatic feeders that feed small amounts throughout the day, lickimats, snuffle pads, etc.

- A cat that is vomiting 1+ times per week raises concern for pathology.

- "Just a hairball" is not considered normal if it is happening often. Yes, hair in vomit = hairball. However, make sure to ask if there are other types of vomit present too. And even if there is hair in the vomitus every time, it is still not "just a hairball" if occurring consistently. This raises concern for pathology due to the inability of the cat to pass hair normally.
    - Note: In short haired cats, frequent vomiting of hairballs can still signify an enteropathy.

STEP 4: Is the underlying cause due to systemic or gastrointestinal disease?

- The first step is to rule out systemic disease. You accomplish this through...

    - Taking a thorough history.
        - Ask about any diet changes?
        - What is the cat vomiting up?
        - When is the cat vomiting?
        - Does the cat eat too quickly and vomit right after?
        - Any other food the cat could be getting into?
        - Any plants in the house? etc.

    - Perform a full physical exam.

    - Perform baseline health screen–see diagnostic plan below.

Some common causes of chronic vomiting in cats

GI Disease	Systemic disease
▶ Food intolerance ▶ Dietary indiscretion ▶ Infection (parasitic, etc.) ▶ Inflammatory bowel disease ▶ Lymphoma or other infiltrative neoplasm ▶ Constipation ▶ Obstruction (bezoars, string or other foreign bodies, etc.) ▽ Check under the tongue in every vomiting cat!	▶ Hyperthyroidism ▶ Kidney/liver disease ▶ Cholangitis ▶ DKA ▶ Pancreatitis ▶ Diaphragmatic hernia ▶ Toxins (flower/plant ingestion, etc.) ▶ Medications ▶ Neurologic (vestibular dz, encephalitis, motion sickness, etc.) ▶ Neoplasia ▶ Stress/fear

STEP 5: Diagnostic plan:

- **Start with routine blood work:** Always start with complete blood work to get a baseline health screen: CBC, chemistry, electrolytes, T4, urinalysis, fecal, +/- FIV/Felv snap test if indicated.

- **Consider imaging or empirical treatment depending on what seems appropriate for the case.** Here are some tips on what we do in certain scenarios...

    - **If the patient is stable and symptoms seem mild or appropriate**, consider starting the empirical treatment plan we outline in the treatment section.
        - For these cases, it is always a good habit to offer imaging early, but let them know that empirical treatment is a reasonable start too. If empirical treatment does not work or the patient worsens at any point, the owner is prepped for the next step of imaging (such as abdominal ultrasound). This allows the owner time to process what you have told them and make the decision as to the next step in a stable patient.

- **Perspective from Dr. Jess:** Empiric treatment (diet change, anti-nausea, slow feeder, etc.) should help in just a couple weeks. If not better, don't wait months until the cat is also very underweight and sick otherwise. Utilize this talking point to push them into performing some diagnostics.

▽ **If your patient is not feeling well, has recently worsened, or has another other reason** you feel seems appropriate to dig deeper (think weight loss, dehydration, etc.), then strongly recommend imaging right away. This helps you tailor an appropriate treatment plan and can guide prognosis. A few notes on imaging...

- **Abdominal ultrasound vs. radiographs:**
  - **Abdominal ultrasound:** It is often the highest yield and a great choice for the long term stable cases. Always warn owners that if one mode of imaging does not find a cause, we may have to consider the other.
    - Example: Dr. Tarantino had an older chronically vomiting cat that had normal blood work and abdominal ultrasound. It was not until x-rays were performed that a chest mass was found and helped guide us to next steps. Point being, they may need both if one does not yield us an answer, and we often recommend both to complete the picture if they can afford it.
  - **Radiographs:** In ill cats, cats with recent worsening of signs, or if ultrasound is unavailable, x-rays are a good place to start. Explain to your owner that x-rays can help screen for obvious causes like an obstruction, diaphragmatic hernia, neoplasia, etc.
- **For owners who approve imaging:** For abnormalities, consider fine needle aspirate or biopsy via endoscopy or abdominal exploratory as ways to gain a definitive diagnosis.
  - **Example:** You find a cat with thickened intestines on ultrasound. Before pursuing a prednisolone trial, a biopsy or aspirate is an ideal next step and can help differentiate between IBD and lymphoma. These tests should be offered (even if owners seem unlikely to pursue, as you will be surprised!), and you can discuss pro's and con's of each with them. Biopsy is preferred, though an aspirate is the least invasive way to try to get an answer. Just warn an owner that an aspirate can come back as non-diagnostic.
  - **Tip from Dr. Jess:** Just remember, when there is diffuse muscularis thickening and moderately enlarged lymph nodes, it can be hard to tell a difference between small cell lymphoma and IBD. It is important

a client knows an FNA may not give an exact answer but can be done the least invasively.

- **For owners who initially decline imaging:** Commonly, these owners come in again when their older cat has lost even more weight. Recommend x-rays and/or abdominal ultrasound again. Explain these tests as a non-invasive way to get a good look at the GI tract and how it will give us a better idea of what is going on internally. Many owners warm up to the idea of further testing over time, so offering testing a second time along with explaining the value can be helpful in persuading an owner.

- If imaging does not yield a diagnosis or help to guide you further, a Texas GI panel (TLI/FpLI/Cobalamin/Folate) can be a good next step to dig deeper.

- Lastly, you can consider trying a treatment plan. See below.

STEP 6: Treatment plan:

1. **Treat underlying systemic disease:** If systemic disease is present, treat the cat for that specific disease.

2. **First line empirical treatments:** If the cat has normal blood work and the owner declines imaging as the next step, or you do not feel imaging is warranted at this time, start empirical treatment. Warn owners if empirical treatment is ineffective, the next step is to reconsider imaging.

    - **Empirical treatment for stable cats with mild symptoms:**
        - **Diet trial:** Your two main options are a GI specific diet or a hydrolyzed diet. Oftentimes, history will help guide you on which one is the best first choice. We will often start with one and then change to the other 3-4 weeks later if the cat is not improving on it. It can take some time to see results, but the key is to tell the owner to expect the cat to steadily improve over time. Prep your owner for this plan.
            - GI specific diet options: Hill's I/D, Purina EN, or Royal Canin GI.
            - Hydrolyzed protein or novel protein options: Hill's Z/D, Purina HA, Royal Canin Ultamino, or Royal Canin PD or PR.
                - If you choose a novel protein option first and find it ineffective, you can consider trying a hydrolyzed diet next. Sometimes one works

better than another. We prefer a hydrolyzed diet, but sometimes picky cats do better with a novel protein.

- ▽ Broad spectrum dewormer such as fenbendazole (50 mg/kg PO for 5 days) or a topical option like Profender (if their cat is a picky eater).
- ▽ Antiemetic such as Cerenia: You can do one injection today or send home with a box of PO tablets for short term use as needed. Just remember, this is treating symptoms and not the underlying disease, so usually this is not an ideal long term plan on its own.
- ▽ +/- probiotic like Purina Fortiflora or Nutramax Proviable.

3. Prednisolone trial: **Always perform blood work and offer/perform imaging prior to doing a prednisolone trial.** We consider prednisolone trials in cases that do not respond to the above or that may have moderate to severe symptoms (See case three below as an example). If owners have declined further imaging, and the cat's blood work, urinalysis, and fecal testing are normal, you have ruled out systemic disease for the most part. Consider a deworming course regardless to be thorough. **Here are a few important notes about prednisolone trials below:**

- ▶ When we do them: If your owner has financial limitations prohibiting imaging on a chronically vomiting cat, and the above empirical treatment is ineffective or the pet is worsening despite this treatment, you can discuss a prednisolone trial.

- ▶ When we have found them most helpful: In our experience, a prednisolone trial can be helpful in your chronically vomiting senior cats where other diseases have been ruled out, and we suspect a high likelihood of GI neoplasia. We have also found it helpful in older cats losing weight with no apparent cause on blood work or imaging.

- ▶ What to have ruled out: Though it is not always possible, we want to make sure we rule out systemic diseases like diabetes, hyperthyroidism, etc. and that we do not suspect a foreign body. In cases where imaging is not an option due to finances, we use our best judgement and caution owners of the risk. Cats with foreign bodies are usually ACUTELY vomiting, inappetent, painful in their abdomen, cannot hold food down, etc.

- ▶ How we do prednisolone trials:
  - ▽ We start with 1.5-2 mg/kg PO total per day for 2 to 4 weeks with the goal of having clinical signs controlled for two straight weeks before gradually tapering dose. Taper dose by ½ until the lowest effective dose is achieved. Some cats only

require tapering courses when symptoms recur, while others need to maintain a low SID or EOD prednisolone dosage long term.

- **Tip from Dr. Jess:** Dividing the dose into BID vs. giving SID does not affect the efficacy of prednisolone. Do whatever dosing is convenient for your client. When tapering, I usually drop by 25% every 2 weeks.
  - **Tapering example:** 10 mg daily for 2 weeks, 7.5 mg daily for 2 weeks, 5 mg daily for 2 weeks, 2.5 mg daily for 2 weeks, and then 2.5 mg every other day for 2 weeks to finish.

- **Example plan with an 8 pound cat:**
  - Prednisolone 5 mg tablet: Give 1 tablet every 12 hours for 2 weeks, then give 1.5 tablets every 24 hours for two weeks. Recheck in 2 weeks with a doctor for recheck weight/assessment/long term plan regarding dosing.

Client communication points prior to prednisolone trial

- First, if at any point they plan to pursue a biopsy in future, the prednisolone trial will affect results, as it can 'mask' the disease. It can also delay wound healing if surgery is needed. This is important for those clients 'on the fence,' so make sure they understand.
- Second, inform them of the risks of diabetes and exacerbating heart disease with chronic steroid use. However, this may be the best option for their cat's comfort and a risk worth taking!
- Third, imaging is strongly preferred, especially due to the adverse side effects of the drug if it is not indicated. An example is if there was a partial obstruction, hernia etc., but if it is truly not an option for the owner, then it is reasonable to still proceed with trial.

4. **Vitamin B12 trial:** An additional treatment to consider, especially if diarrhea is present also.

   a. See chronic diarrhea chapter for more information as well as reference the Texas A&M protocols.

5. **Other treatment considerations:** If your prednisolone trial does not work, re-evaluate if new diagnostics should be pursued or repeated. In presumptive IBD/GI lymphoma cases refractory to prednisolone, chlorambucil can be added in. Before doing this, you will want to have had some sort of imaging as well as a frank discussion of risks and monitoring requirements. As with prednisolone, you taper to the lowest effective dose. With chlorambucil you should also be checking a CBC at 2-4 weeks initially, then 6-8 weeks and finally every 3-6 months ongoing, to look for any signs of myelosuppression.

Three common chronic vomiting examples and treatment plans

1. **Example one: Healthy cat at a yearly exam that is vomiting biweekly.**

   An example is a middle aged DSH cat that shows up for a yearly exam with a history of biweekly vomiting for months or even years. The owner insists they are just hairballs, but when you ask if hair is always in it, the answer is no. No weight loss or other abnormal findings are noted on the exam.

Never forget this...from Dr. Jess

Get a weight! It should be standard, but if a cat is spicy or it's a tight appointment, it is often the first thing to be missed. Weight trending is critical in chronic GI cases and builds cases for "we have to do something more" when you can catch subtle loss.

   a. **Convincing these owners that their cat's vomiting is abnormal can be tough in some cases.** These owners have become accustomed to it and see vomiting as a normal symptom of their cat.
      i. If you feel the **cat is stable, recommend a complete blood work panel** mentioned above and explain how a cat's health can change year to year. This is a minimally invasive way to be thorough for a baseline health screen. With a stable patient, you can send the blood work out and call in a few days.

   b. **If blood work comes back within normal limits,** you should have a heart to heart with the owner to explain how there still could be disease present based on such a high frequency of vomiting. Reinforce the idea that frequent vomiting in cats is not normal. Frequent hairballs are not normal either, even for long-haired cats. Explain that you have many options that can be tried over the next 3-6 months, and the goal is to decrease vomiting frequency as much as possible. Otherwise, further diagnostics may be needed to dig deeper and continue the search for the underlying cause.

c. **Easy first options** for an owner unwilling to dig deeper with diagnostics include:
    i. **Recommend a diet change to a prescription diet for at least 3-4 weeks** to assess response to therapy. Roll through each option to see what works for their cat. Remember to tell your clients to go slowly with transitions to avoid diarrhea, refusal, etc. **We like this advice:** 75% old 25% new for a few days, 50% of each for a few days, and then by day 7-10 you are at 75% new 25% old and finally by 2-3 weeks you are at 100% new.
        1. **Option one** is aimed at treating a food allergy, inflammatory bowel disease, etc.
            a. Hypoallergenic diets such as Hill's Z/D, Purina HA, or Royal Canin Ultamino.
        2. **Option two** is a GI diet, which is highly digestible and prebiotics that can benefit generic digestive issues.
            a. Hill's I/D, Purina EN, or Royal Canin gastroenteric.
            b. If the cat is having diarrhea too, consider a fiber forward diet like Hill's GI Biome or add fiber to these diets (chia seeds, psyllium, fiber one, etc.); See chronic diarrhea chapter for more information.
        3. **Option three** is to try a novel protein diet. It can be used when someone is unwilling to purchase a prescription diet or wants an option they can pick up from a store more easily. It also may be more palatable if a cat won't eat a hypoallergenic diet.
        4. **Note:** If the client is unwilling to buy a prescription product, consider other over the counter options like Purina Pro Plan sensitive stomach, stopping added treats, switching to a slow feeder bowl, and even a trial of strictly wet food (if previously on dry...or vice versa). Some cats respond to these simple changes, especially if the owner is changing food and treats routinely. Warn these owners, that if this does not improve vomiting that a prescription diet trial will still be needed.

ii. **Send home a broad spectrum dewormer.** We like a 5 day course of fenbendazole. Another easy option if you have a picky cat is topical Profender (one treatment).

iii. **For cats with hairball issues or extremely long haired cats:** Ensure that they are brushing their cat often (at least a few times per week) and/or are getting them shaved so that they can prevent progressive issues like an obstruction.

   1. Dr. Gray has a long-haired cat who has a hairball issue. He will start to decrease his appetite around the time of a hairball getting large so it provides a clue something is coming. Since he is not amenable to regular brushing, she gets him sedated and shaved down 1-2 times per year to try to help this issue.

Client communication summary for a healthy yearly cat with chronic vomiting

- Start by asking questions and characterizing vomiting.
- Know that often these owners have grown accustomed to their cat vomiting and see it as "normal."
- Explain that this is not normal and even though their cat looks good, we need to look into it further.
- Easy place to start is screening blood work and fecal testing.
- Reasonable, inexpensive treatment plan to start with is a diet change and dewormer.
- Let them know that at some point if the vomiting persists, more diagnostics will need to be done such as abdominal ultrasound to get more information.

2. Example two: **Sick cat of any age that is vomiting.**

   An example is a DMH cat of any age that presents with chronic intermittent vomiting over the last three weeks. History notes lethargy, sudden weight loss, hyporexia, and dehydration. These cats will present as appointments or walk-ins emergencies, and many can appear unstable on physical exam.

   a. Perform a thorough physical looking for a string under the tongue, pale or icteric gums, palpate for a large colon or abdominal pain, make sure there are no signs of a urinary obstruction, .etc. You have to go through our basic approach to be thorough and ensure you start the appropriate diagnostics and treatment.

   b. **Cats that present sick benefit from all diagnostics.** Prioritize in house blood work and thoracic/abdominal x-rays. You want to get as much information as possible to rule out concerning causes that could require aggressive therapy or surgery.

   c. **Do not be afraid to start treatments right away if the cat's clinical status concerns you and an owner is on board to be thorough today.** Consider giving the cat some subcutaneous fluids, an anti-nausea medication, or even placing an IV catheter for IV fluids while you await your results. As you get your results back, you can determine if your cat can have outpatient care vs. hospitalization vs. referral vs. other.
      i. Tip from Dr. Jess: Remember that anti-nausea medications can mask more significant issues, so don't send home oral without ruling out an obstruction first. Tell an owner that if they vomit through a good anti-nausea medication (like Cerenia), it is a sign something significant is going on, and they need to come back or go to the ER. You also want to make sure the patient is not on any NSAIDs so be thorough in your medication history taking.

Client communication summary for a sick cat of any age that is vomiting

- Perform a thorough physical exam (We give you clues of things to look for above.).
- Let owners know that with the signs of illness and physical exam findings you are very concerned and feel strongly that both blood work and x-rays will be warranted. You should also consider checking a UA and fecal based on results.
- Consider inpatient vs. outpatient therapy depending on severity, findings, and financial ability.
- Set up a long term management plan when appropriate.

3. Example three: **Older cat that is "stable" with weight loss and vomiting.**

An example is a geriatric cat that presents during an annual exam with the mention of vomiting that is made in passing. Other times, they are brought in for a sick visit because of weight loss.

a. It is really important to start our basic approach to rule out underlying systemic disease like diabetes, hyperthyroidism, etc. You have the option of doing blood work out house or in house based on if you, or the owner, feels it is important to get answers that day.

b. This weight loss may have been going on for a long time (weeks to months), so just use your best judgement based on your exam as to if this cat needs diagnostics today or if you can wait a few days. If the cat feels dehydrated with decreased skin turgor, looks unthrifty, or emaciated, then you can suggest doing it in house because of these factors. Give the owner the option.

c. Warn these owners that you may not find a cause on blood work, so the next step is imaging. By mentioning this early, you are prepping your owner, and many are open to performing imaging when they have had time to process everything.

d. If you find diagnostics to be unremarkable and the owner declines imaging due to cost, then move forward with the empirical therapy mentioned above +/- prednisolone trial +/- vitamin B12 injections. Start step by step and have follow up phone calls and rechecks planned so that you can tailor treatment to response.

i. Be sure to explain to the owner that we still have options here despite diagnostics. It is important to warn your owner of the side effects of treating this way without a diagnosis. However, the only other option is continued weight loss which we do not want either. If the owner cannot afford a prescription diet, we prioritize the prednisolone trial, dewormer, vitamin B12 injections, and then diet.
    1. **Tip from Dr. Jess:** She strongly recommends getting a baseline B12 prior to starting it because you lose the chance to evaluate it later as a diagnostic tool. You might be signing them up for a treatment they don't need, so look into what a B12 test costs if the client is not willing to do a full Texas GI panel.

ii. Also, do not forget to go through the client communication points on prednisolone trials with owners mentioned in the treatment section above!

Client communication summary for an older 'stable' cat with weight loss and vomiting

- Discuss the weight loss and PE findings as well as the importance of starting to look for underlying systemic disease.
- Start with blood work and urinalysis (in house or send out as you feel fit) and let owners know that if you do not find a cause, then the next step is x-rays and abdominal ultrasound.
- If owners decline imaging, consider starting empirical treatment like diet change, dewormer, pred trial, +/- vitamin B12. See client communication summary on pred trials in previous section.
- In older cats with weight loss, we do not wait as long to get to the pred trial as we would with the relatively healthy cats that come in with vomiting (as seen in case one).
- Be sure to rule out diabetes prior to a pred trial!

NOTES:

NOTES:

Cushing's Disease in Dogs

Reviewed by Dr. Jessica Romine, DVM, DACVIM

You will have many patients come in to see you with clinical signs that SCREAM Cushing's disease. Yet many of these patients will still test negative for it! It can be a difficult disease to diagnose! We find that it can take time to develop in some patients, so fear not, and just prepare your owner that you may need to retest in the near future. Ensure your owner understands that while it is a fairly common endocrine disease in dogs, it is one that is important to diagnose correctly before treatment. We are here to talk you through everything from diagnosis to treatment options to pertinent client communication points. PLUS, there are two bonus chapters at the end on how to discuss ALKP elevations with your clients and how to perform an ACTH stimulation test.

Some common presentations you will see

- **Older pet with PU/PD and an elevation of ALKP +/- pot bellied appearance, skin issues, lethargy, excessive panting, etc.**
    - ▽ **Example:** 12 year old MN dog with rotund abdomen, fragile looking skin, and has a 'bad knee'. He has dilute urine on UA and an elevated ALKP. Owner says he has always drunk a lot of water, but they do not think it is more than normal. Test this patient!
- **Older pet with non-resolving skin issues, pot bellied abdomen, pants excessively, and an elevated ALKP.**
    - ▽ **Example:** 10 year old FS dog with hair falling out in clumps. She has an elevated ALKP, normal thyroid levels, and a USG in the 'gray zone' (1.012-1.018). The owner says she has always drank a lot of water, and she inappropriately urinates in the house sometimes because of it. Test this patient!
- **You get the gist!**

When do you test for Cushing's disease?

In general, we do not test for Cushing's disease just because of an elevation of ALKP alone. We test patients with clinical signs of Cushing's disease noted on exam and appropriate symptoms noted at home. First, make sure you have ruled out other diseases like a urinary tract infection, hypothyroidism, liver disease, kidney disease, etc. Then, you can dive into testing options.

Reminder from Dr. Jess

Remember that our Cushing's testing is based on evaluating chronic cortisol elevations in the blood, so anything that would do this can interfere, including any non-adrenal illness, chronic stress at home, and administration of exogenous steroids (including oral, ocular and aural formulations!). If the patient is on these, it will be difficult to interpret results.

The basics of diagnosis

It is ideal to get two tests that indicate Cushing's disease is present, but it is not necessary. One positive test is enough to start treatment. Dr. Jess wants to humanize that this disease is SO not straightforward compared to what they teach you in school, and as an internist she has had many patients that scream Cushing's but test negative with various presentations. Remember that the adrenals produce non-cortisol hormones as well (sex hormones) that have similar effects and that we're testing cortisol levels in sick animals. Warn people that it can be a real rigamarole to get an answer in some cases. In human medicine, they get a CT scan/MRI to look at their pituitary and a full adrenal panel (cortisol, sex hormones, aldosterone, etc) to look for Cushing's. We don't have the ability to go to that diagnostic level in all our cases so we do the best we can!

1. **Blood test (LDDST and ACTH stim test):** We often will start with one of these tests (usually the LDDST) though there are pros and cons to both and each case must be evaluated individually. The **low dose dexamethasone suppression test (LDDST)** is the ACVIM test of choice for non-iatrogenic Cushing's based on their 2012 consensus statement. It picks up on 90% of Cushing's patients and also allows you to rule in or out PDH about 50% of the time. You can certainly do the **ACTH stimulation test** to diagnose Cushing's if you prefer it

instead. It has less false positives and is faster to perform. We typically choose the ACTH stim test over LDDST if the pet is sick or has diabetes. Iatrogenic Cushing's can usually be ruled out with a good history. You will want to stop the medication causing the side effects in these cases and get it out of the system before re-evaluating this patient.

a. There are pros and cons to each, and if we do not trust findings on one of these tests, we may pursue abdominal ultrasound or run the other test.

b. You will also use your ACTH stim test to monitor medication dosage at recheck visits. You do not need to have a baseline ACTH stim test prior to starting medication if you have a positive LDDST.

2. **Urine Cortisol:Creatinine Ratio** (Dr. Jess loves this test, and here's why!): This can be a good screening test, especially if you don't have a high suspicion: think only a high ALP and/or if a dog is hard to get blood on.

    a. This test is very sensitive (i.e. if it is negative, it is probably not Cushing's) but not specific.

    b. It is important to have the owners bring in a urine sample a few days after the vet visit. The excitement of the exam can falsely elevate it. You should also not perform it if the dog is sick with other things.

3. **Abdominal ultrasound** is a good test to perform before or after your blood test.

    a. The reason is that it gets you a full health screen on the pet by assessing all other organs, and you can assess adrenal gland size.

        i. Dr. Jess wanted to share that up to 25% of patients can have normal adrenal glands and still have Cushing's disease. Many larger breed dogs (especially Labs) can have adrenal hyperplasia so don't use ultrasound as a hard and fast test. Even if they don't do surgery, it's still relevant to know if they have an adrenal tumor to contend with or PDH.

    b. Some pets will have a severely enlarged adrenal gland (one or both), which could indicate a benign or malignant neoplasm is present and can allow you to determine if PDH vs. ADH, if the LDDST test did not tell you.

i. From Dr. Jess: If you find an adrenal tumor, consider urine metanephrine testing, especially if your patient doesn't scream Cushing's otherwise, as pheos can also raise ALP.

c. See below for a few scenarios where we feel this is the most important first step.

d. If the owner cannot afford an abdominal ultrasound, we will go forward with treatment based on a blood test (LDDST or ACTH stim test) in support of the disease and appropriate clinical signs. If you are ever unsure and need guidance, it can be very helpful to consult with an internal medicine specialist from the lab who ran your sample (Idexx or Antech) for advice on treatment. It is free!

When to postpone Cushing's testing and do an abdominal ultrasound first

- **A sick animal.** First, we need to clarify what we mean by sick in this example. We are talking about animals that are not feeling well (lethargic, not eating well, etc.). We are NOT talking about animals that have signs of Cushing's disease but still feel relatively well (have PU/PD, panting, skin infections etc.). Technically, you CAN test for Cushing's if you want on a lethargic, inappetent dog. **However, with sick animals, it could be something else making them feel ill. You should start by being thorough and looking into all the reasons why they may be sick with blood work, urinalysis, and imaging, etc.**
    - In general, we do not start pets that are sick on Trilostane or Mitotane. These medications can have side effects, particularly with gastrointestinal upset and anorexia, so we want them to feel better before starting these medications.
        - From Dr. Jess: Cushing's is chronic and doesn't usually cause major GI upset, inappetence, or lethargy, so it shouldn't be making them ill unless it's triggered by something else. Examples of other concurrent diseases could be high blood pressure/stroke, diabetes, gallbladder mucocele, etc. If that's happening, you need to address that disease first anyway.
    - If needed, ACTH stimulation test is the test we would do here because it is more accurate in sick patients than LDDST and can help you rule out Addison's too, which can be a cause of sick, lethargic dogs.

- **Apparently healthy dog with just an ALKP elevation:** 7 year old FS dog that is apparently healthy and has an ALKP of 600 that has been climbing slowly over the last few years. Let the owner know about the increase over time and that the rest of her blood work looks great. Ultrasound is offered to the owner who wants more information as a way to look into possible reasons why it may be climbing. It is important to stress that ultrasound may show nothing, but it will allow us to rule out many causes and feel better with our monitoring and treatment plan.
  - **Tip from Dr. Jess:** I usually consider running triglycerides on these patients as hypertriglyceridemia (Cushing's or on its own) can drive vacuolar hepatopathy/ high ALP and is easily treatable.

Tips on LDDST and ACTH stim test

- If the pet is not on therapy, they should be fasted because lipemia can interfere with results.
- However, if a pet did eat, you can fast them for 4-6 hours at the clinic, then do the test.
- Water does not interfere with results.
- If the dog is already on Trilostane, they should be given a small meal the day of the test because Trilostane works best absorbed with food.

Client communication summary for Cushing's

- Brief explanation of the disease, complications of unregulated disease and the prognosis.
- Explain the commitment needed to manage this disease with medication. Emphasize a team approach.
- Discuss medication and risks associated with them and what they can expect.
- Discuss expected costs (medications, initial testing and long term management costs).
- Discuss possible complications and signs to watch out for (adrenal necrosis, joint pain, etc.).

1. **Cushing's disease basics:**

- What it is: Communicate to your owner that Cushing's disease means that their pet has an excessive amount of cortisol being produced. It is either due to a tumor in the pituitary gland of their brain (majority) or an adrenal gland tumor. These can invade the vena cava, so sometimes surgery is recommended. Typically, these adrenal tumors are malignant (carcinoma) and pituitary tumors are benign. If the adrenal glands are enlarged from a pituitary tumor (due to being overstimulated-like how a muscle gets big from exercise), they can have implications on the body such as delayed healing, more prone to injury (such as cranial cruciate ligament rupture), infections (typically skin and urinary as most common), hypertension, clot formation (stroke-like events), and overall unhealthy dogs if we do not treat them. These health risks will be reduced with good control of the disease. **The goal of treatment is reducing clinical signs, maintaining quality of life and decreasing possibility of problems from unregulated Cushing's.**
    - **Tip from Dr. Jess:** 10% of the time dogs with the pituitary form will develop neurologic signs (seizures, personality change, etc.) because of the tumor growing large, even though it's benign. Anecdotally I see this more in my Staffies and middle- to large-sized dogs over little dogs, but it can happen to any!

- Prognosis: Typically, prognosis is good. Most signs will disappear quickly, while others will improve over time. If a patient has concurrent disease (such as Diabetes), it can be more difficult to regulate them well.
    - **For those who are on the fence about treating...some data from Dr. Jess to share!:** In general, treating Cushing's extends survival vs. not. Some owners aren't bothered by the clinical signs of PU/PD, alopecia, etc. so they do not feel highly motivated to treat. This is absolutely fine, but if they ask if it is harmful to the dog, you can share "no not directly, but a study has shown it can shorten their lifespan over time."
        - Lifespan research: Seventeen dogs received trilostane, and 26 received no treatment. By the date of censoring (death or 2 years after diagnosis), 6 (35%) of the dogs in the trilostane group and 17 (65%) of the dogs in the untreated group had died. Two-year survival rates were 52.2% in the trilostane group and 8.5% in the untreated group. The median survival time (at which half the dogs were dead) was not reached for the trilostane group because more than half were still alive at the time of censoring. **Median survival in the untreated group was 506 days (95% CI, 292–564 days), significantly shorter than in the trilostane group.** 2017

- Also Schofield I, Brodbelt DC, Wilson ARL, Niessen S, Church D, O'Neill D. Survival analysis of 219 dogs with hyperadrenocorticism attending primary care practice in England. Vet Rec. 2020 Mar 21;186(11):348. doi: 10.1136/vr.105159. Epub 2019 Sep 20. PMID: 31542726; PMCID: PMC7146928.

- **The commitment:** Cushing's disease is a manageable disease and one that we feel owners can see a great improvement in quality of life. Though, it is important they are aware of the commitment. There is a commitment to being diligent with medication, communicating any concerns to the doctor, and coming in for rechecks when recommended. It is not a disease that can be managed well if rechecks are forgotten. We let owners know that quality of life with this disease is possible and is the main goal of treatment. It is also something that requires commitment from owners.

- **Medication options and risks:** Our treatment of choice is Trilostane. This drug is the safest of the two and the only FDA approved drug to treat both pituitary and adrenal-dependent Cushing's disease in dogs.

    - **Trilostane** is a synthetic steroid analogue that interferes in the pathway of cortisol production.

    - **Mitotane** is a human chemotherapy drug used off label, and it can have more serious side effects due to the potential for causing Addison's disease from destruction of the adrenal gland.

    - We let owners know that both drugs are very serious, but most pets do well with them. We warn them of the risks. There is risk of sudden death with Trilostane, though that is VERY rare. There is also a risk of adrenal necrosis with Trilostane, which is uncommon but can occur anytime while on the medication (hence why we recommend regular ACTH stimulation testing). This is why, no matter what treatment the owner's elect, we make a big deal of them paying CLOSE ATTENTION to their dog's DAILY mood, appetite, energy level, etc. ACTH stimulation tests should be repeated anytime pets show any signs of illness or being off. We advise owners not to 'wait and see' if signs resolve while on these medications.

- ▽ Always mention to owners and look for signs of the opposite disease, Addison's disease, such as anorexia +/- vomiting, diarrhea, etc.
    - ➔ Dr. Jess tip: Generally, it is recommended for owners to skip a dose of Trilostane if their dog is not eating or feeling well when the dose is due, even if it is a clinical sign from other causes. They could probably benefit from a little extra cortisol on those days.

- ▽ ****If they even pause before eating when they are normally a food hound, we want to know about it!****
    - ➔ That is one sign that has allowed us to catch doses that were too high on what we had perceived to be well regulated Cushing's patients.

- ▽ If you emphasize their task to call and bring the pet in if they notice any oddities, then you will be able to work well together as a team to make sure they are doing well on these strong drugs. Our goal is not to scare owners with this but to help them understand the importance of being vigilant to prevent issues with treatment.

2. **Expected costs:**

- ▶ Let them know the cost of the medication. It can be pricey for larger dogs.

- ▶ Initial testing period: **ACTH stimulation testing is performed 2-4 weeks after starting the medication** to assess response to therapy. Then, sometimes 1 or 2 more times during the adjustment phase in the first 2-3 months until you feel they are appropriately regulated. Warn an owner that if we have difficulty regulating their pet, this may require a specialist second opinion. Let the owner know the average cost of an ACTH stimulation test, so they are not caught off guard at recheck visits. (For us, it is around $200-300 due to the high cost of Cortrosyn.)
    - ▽ **Tip from Dr. Jess:** Pre-pill cortisol monitoring is also acceptable now in many cases.
        - ➔ Here is a protocol (Australian, but rules are the same): https://www.gribblesvets.com.au/media/1533/updates-in-the-management-of-canine-hyperadrenocorticism-2.pdf
            - ↓ Important to know about pre-pill cortisol monitoring: It is less expensive since you're only doing one cortisol measurement, and you don't need Synacthen. However, it must be done in the morning BEFORE the morning dose (and if they get the meds once a day in the

evening, then BEFORE that dose!). It's appropriate for dogs that are doing well, and only if there is a concern they may be over-dosed, an ACTH stimulation is appropriate to rule out hypoadrenocorticism instead. You also need to interpret in context. If you get a pre-pill cortisol that's a little low, but the dog is reported to be doing great, you don't always have to drop down on the dosage. This is where it's an art and not just a science.

- **A source to check out:** https://pmc.ncbi.nlm.nih.gov/articles/PMC5256409/

- **Long term testing:** Once their pet is **well regulated, we like to do an ACTH stimulation test every 3 to 6 months** when on a good dose to ensure they are maintaining well. Routine blood work with blood pressure will also be performed every 6-12 months to keep tabs on overall health.
    - If a client cannot afford all of these tests in the long term monitoring phase, focus on clinical signs to guide you and consider a pre-pill cortisol level in lieu of ACTH Stim (usually 12-24 hours after a dose of Trilostane). Always caution owner's with financial restraints of importance of routine testing (because of adrenal necrosis) and set up a plan within reason they can adhere too.

3. **Short term complications:**

- Most commonly, you will find that some dogs get transient GI upset (vomiting, diarrhea) or anorexia.

- If this occurs, you can prescribe medications to manage these clinical signs and/or consider a dose adjustment. This may mean lowering your dosage or going to every other day dosing for 2-3 weeks to give their body time to adjust to the medication.

4. **Long term complications:**

- It is important to emphasize that their dog has an endocrine disease and may be prone to other diseases like high blood pressure. **With this disease, it will be very important that we keep tabs on any signs of illness, and if they are noted, we recommend bringing them in right away.** Their pet may not be able to ward off illnesses and can be more prone to getting sick than when they were younger and healthier.

- When these dogs are not feeling well, one of the first things we do is an ACTH stimulation test. Adrenal gland necrosis can still occur with Trilostane and is a complication that can make these pets very sick. This complication is NOT dose-dependent, so it can happen at any time (though it is still very rare!).

5. **Medication choice: Trilostane or Mitotane?**

    - Trilostane is the drug of choice (FDA approved), but both can be used reasonably well. Trilostane may be cost prohibitive for some owners, and Mitotane is fairly affordable. In full transparency, neither of us has experience with Mitotane. We tend to stick to FDA approved medications whenever they are available. Both require routine monitoring, as mentioned above. We will focus on Trilostane (most common) here. It can be compounded if needed.

        - **Trilostane therapy: 2 mg/kg PO SID in the am with food OR 1 mg/kg PO BID with food**
            - Dr. Jess tip: If your client can afford it, twice daily dosing is more effective at controlling signs. You can also use lower total doses with twice daily dosing.
                - **Dr. Jess tip:** If a client can manage it financially, dosing trilostane twice daily tends to do a better job of controlling clinical signs, since the medication usually only lasts about 8–10 hours. Using a twice-daily schedule also allows for lower total doses, and when a patient is borderline between doses, it's best to err on the lower side. This approach is especially important for dogs with diabetes, as controlling cortisol for only part of the day can make blood sugar harder to regulate. Trilostane should always be given with food to improve its absorption.
            - ACTH stimulation test is used to monitor patients once therapy is started (see chart at end of book for how to perform). We test 2-4 weeks after starting Trilostane. You want to perform it 4-6 hours after the Trilostane dose was given with food. For reliable testing, Trilostane must be given with food because it is fat soluble. Try to time your patient's test around the same time as previously done to get comparable results.
                - As mentioned above, you can also consider Pre-pill cortisol monitoring. See earlier in the chapter for details and a link for more information.

- Test anywhere from 2-4 weeks after dose adjustments are made. We generally test one more time at 3 months after we stabilize, if finances allow.
- Always assess clinical signs and weight when you are checking if a dose change is warranted.
- Long term, we perform an ACTH stimulation test every 4-6 months once stabilized.

▽ Once we start a dog on Trilostane therapy, we often find that initially the values are still a bit higher than we want. Most of the time, we ***still keep the patient on the same dose and resist the urge to put them on a higher dose, unless clinical signs are unchanged.*** This is because over the first 1-3 months, their body is acclimating to the drug. Trilostane can become more effective over time. You can run the risk of overdosing them if you increase the dose after their first follow-up test. This holds true throughout the course of the disease, as even over time pets can be more 'sensitive' to the initial dose of Trilostane. This is why we still perform regular ACTH stim tests, as your patient may continue to need dose adjustments in the future.

Timing for improvement of clinical signs

From Dr. Jess

- PU/PD improves within 1-3 weeks of getting good control
- Hunger and panting improves within 2-4 weeks
- Skin can take months to improve, and coat can get worse initially, as dead hair in the telogenic phase cycles out. The first seasonal shed usually starts to come in better.
- Unfortunately, Cushing's myopathy often doesn't significantly improve

- Always find out if clinical signs are improving and consult with the Idexx or Antech internal medicine specialist for help if you are unsure what to do. A good rule of thumb is that if your patient is still out of the reference range and has no improvement in clinical signs, then you can increase their dosage a small amount. If you opt to keep the same dose due to clinical signs improving, then plan to test again in 1-3 months. Once stabilized, testing will back off to every 4-6 months with retesting ~4 weeks after dose changes.

One side effect of treating Cushing's disease is joint pain!

We want to discuss a quick side note with you as something we have noticed in practice. When you have a patient with a high dose of cortisol flowing through their bloodstream, it keeps inflammation down. This applies to our older patients who have arthritis that have been benefiting greatly from said cortisol levels. When we take this away from them, they often start showing signs of pain because all of a sudden they do not have this anti-inflammatory effect of cortisol. We mention this to owners, and then will often communicate that once we get them regulated, we may need to start them on medications like joint supplements and NSAIDs. It is important to note here too that if a pet parent chooses not to treat Cushing's disease, it can put the dog at higher risk for cruciate ruptures. Steroids weaken those ligaments, so ensure they pay attention to their pet's mobility (or lack there of) to help guide treatment options. See our osteoarthritis chapter for more information!

Final points

Cushing's disease can be fairly straightforward to manage. However, in order for it to go smoothly, we try to keep the following in mind:

- If possible, try to get an abdominal ultrasound in addition to a blood test before treating your patient.
- Know and mention the cost of treatment to your client, as the medications can be expensive. Ensure they understand it is not curative, but rather managed with medications.
- Wait to treat until you are sure it is truly Cushing's disease. The medications are serious, so you need to ensure the owner understands this and the importance of a thorough work-up.
    - **Tip from Dr. Jess:** Compounding Trilostane is NOT a good option to fit dose sizes or to make it cheaper. They are unreliable. In this paper, of the 44 trilostane-containing packets, only 40.9% (18 packets) had acceptable strength of Trilostane in them.
        - Nam S, Kim T, Song K, Feldman EC, Seo K. Evaluation of compounded trilostane packets for dogs with naturally occurring hyperadrenocorticism. J Vet Intern Med. 2021;35(4):1729-1732. doi:10.1111/jvim.16197. Accessed January 21, 2026. https://www.ncbi.nlm.nih.gov/pmc/articles/PMC8295693
- Ensure owners understand this is a disease that requires diligent monitoring and rechecks with you due to the seriousness of the medication.
- Mention common side effects of the drugs to owners: reduced or poor appetite, vomiting, lack of energy, diarrhea, and weakness so they can alert you if noted.
- You must ensure the owner has an understanding of what signs to look out for that could indicate the dog is not feeling well once you begin treatment. The more severe signs, though rare, an owner may see are collapse, severe electrolyte imbalances, and destruction of the adrenal gland (could result in death).

NOTES:

NOTES:

NOTES:

Cutaneous Mast Cell Tumor in Dogs

Reviewed by Dr. Jeff Tinsley, DVM, DACVD

Mast cell tumors are the most common skin tumor in dogs (account for about 20% of what you see). This is one of the few masses you can easily diagnose via in-house cytology. These malignant skin tumors often follow the classic presentation you learned in school, but there are a lot of different things you need to remember when managing these cases. We are going to discuss in detail some of the common presentations you will encounter, exam tips, treatment plans, different grades, and more.

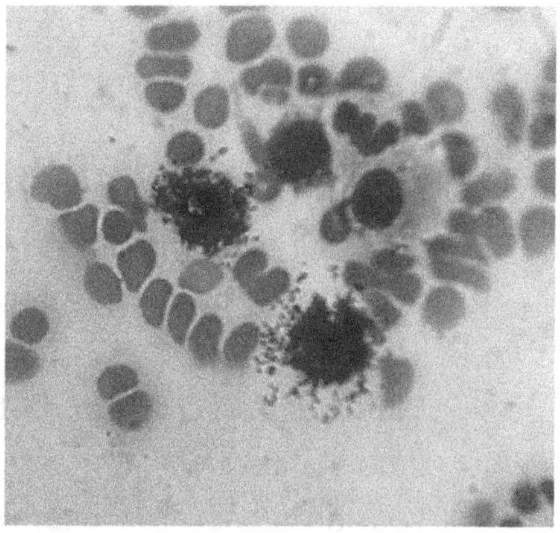

The basics

Presentation: Commonly, you will hear an owner say that a mass has suddenly popped up on their dog's skin and is rapidly changing size (either continuing to grow or waxing/waning in size). There are some that slowly grow though, so do not be fooled. This is one of the few times you can actually believe an owner when they say "Doc, it just popped up overnight!" **ALWAYS OFFER CYTOLOGY ON A NEW MASS (If they say no, document it).**

- **Common signalment:** Most common breeds to develop a mast cell tumor are your brachycephalic dogs like Bulldogs, Boxers, Pugs, etc., and Retriever breeds. However, they can still be seen in any dog.
    - ▽ **Side note:** Unfortunately, we can see them in young and old dogs. Dr. Gray's family Golden Retriever had her first mast cell tumor around the age of 1, so do

not get fooled by age and chalk it up to being a histiocytoma (common benign pretender that mimics a mast cell tumor).

- **Appearance:** These vary significantly from a raised mass above or below the skin to an area that is red, swollen, or ulcerated. We have seen them vary in size from a few millimeters to centimeters.

- **Location:** You will commonly see these masses on the skin (can be anywhere!). 50-60% of them are found on the trunk (neck, thorax, lumbar region) and 15-20% on the limbs. Do not forget that they can also be systemic affecting certain organs (spleen, liver, gastrointestinal tract, bone marrow, etc.). When they metastasize, we often see them travel to the local lymph nodes, spleen, and liver. Rarely, they could go to the lungs.

    - Note: Those that are on the muzzle, mucocutaneous junctions, inguinal, scrotal, perineal, or preputial region tend to be more aggressive. When you find them here, it may be worth a phone call to an oncologist for planning or referral purposes.

- **Clinical signs:** Oftentimes, there are none. However, you can sometimes see pruritus, swelling, redness, or gastrointestinal signs (vomiting, diarrhea, ulceration). Rarely, you can get severe systemic signs like hypotension and SIRS.

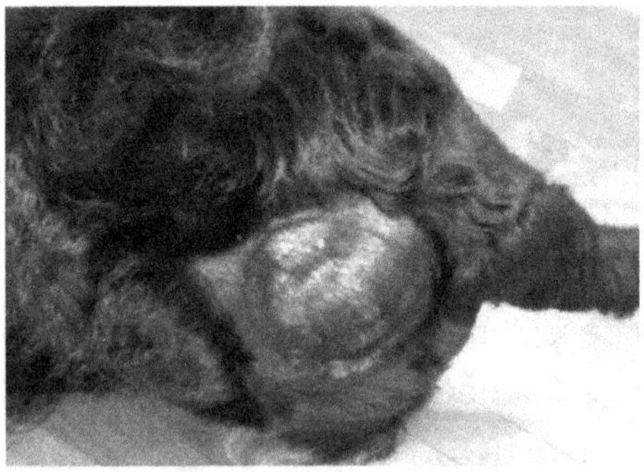

Tip: **The 'mast cell that mimics': Some mast cell tumors LOOK AND FEEL LIKE LIPOMAS. This mast cell tumor almost fooled Dr. Gray. It could have been a lipoma with how it looked and felt.** The fact that it grew VERY rapidly concerned her, so she did cytology that day. This is why you ALWAYS recommend cytology, friends! You can get fooled when they do not have the textbook appearance. **Reminder from Dr. Jeff: Palpation of a suspect "lipoma" is never a substitute for diagnostics. Fine needle aspiration is quick and easy!** If you are running behind, don't let this be a barrier to care. You can always collect the samples, make your slides, and have your support team stain them for you. If your client is unable to wait (because typically we find these appointments go beyond 30 minutes), let them know you will call with the results and can discuss a plan over the phone. Anything beyond a benign mass will typically require a follow-up staging/diagnostic visit anyways, and you cannot do everything in one 30 minute visit. Protect your time and peace by setting boundaries here and being open with the client so they know their options.

Your plan at the initial exam:

Perform the 7 below steps during your initial exam:

1. Measure.
2. Look for others, and perform a thorough physical exam.
3. Cytology in house (send out if uncertain).
4. Diphenhydramine Injection once diagnosed.
5. Start patient on famotidine, diphenhydramine, omeprazole +/- prednisone.
6. Client communication: It is not a one size fits all situation. Lower grades can be curative with surgery if you are able to get margins, while higher grades may need referral. Biopsy will tell you the grade, and additional diagnostics are indicated to look for metastasis.
7. Do baseline lab work if the owner is amenable to surgery.

Initial exam: Please, for the love of vet med, ALWAYS measure your masses. Calipers are cheap, and you can keep them in your pocket. Some owners will decline diagnostics, so by keeping track of measurements, you can easily assess if a mass is rapidly changing over time or remaining stable. Some owners are more willing to perform cytology at the next visit if you can tell them it has grown 2 centimeters in 2 months. Look for others on the pet, and perform a complete dermatologic and physical exam.

Diagnostics: Perform a fine needle aspirate for in-house cytology. Use one of the below two techniques to collect your samples, whichever makes you more comfortable. Typically, your smaller, fragile masses (<5-6 mm) respond best to the woodpecker technique, but the goal is to ensure you get the best representation of the mass. Microscopically, you will see many mast cells throughout your slide +/- purple granules scattered in the background. Ask a fellow DVM to check behind your cytology to build your confidence, and you can even keep a cytology atlas near the microscope for quick reference and when in doubt, send it out!

- **Pro-tip from Dr. Jeff:** Save yourself an extra slide when you perform FNAs. As you diagnose new tumors, you can create a personalized, labeled slide deck for yourself. Even if you send out samples to a pathologist, make sure you have an extra, labeled slide for your collection. As you get more confirmed diagnoses, you can update your personalized slides and BOOM you can reference your own work! Then you will feel more confident over time as the collection builds. As long as you use cover slips, your collection can last an extremely long time. Some clinicians even glue coverslips onto great, diagnostic slides that may keep for years.

1. The **woodpecker method** is a good technique where you take a 22 gauge needle and insert it in and out of a mass in multiple directions to get some cells. You then attach the needle to a 6 mL syringe (plunger already extended) and aspirate the contents onto a slide. To get the most cells, detach the needle, extend the plunger, re-attach the needle and repeat the process 1-2 more times.

2. You can also aspirate using the **classic method** of a 6 mL syringe with a 22g needle attached that is then inserted into the mass. Next disconnect the needle, pull back the plunger to fill the syringe with air, and re-attach the needle to aspirate the sample onto your slide. It is very important to never pull the plunger back while your sampled needle is attached as your precious, precious cells can easily get trapped in the syringe!

Side note: We have both had a few cytologies where we see a few mast cells on the slide, but there are other cell populations in higher numbers. Those often come back as reactive/inflammatory, so a good rule of thumb is that MCT will often have many mast cells noted throughout the slide. We still suggest sending these out as a precaution if it is not clear cut.

When you aspirate a mass that is concerning for MCT, tell the owner to monitor the area/pet closely while you are performing your cytology. Sometimes, the above clinical signs occur after an aspirate due to degranulation. **Once a MCT is diagnosed, go ahead and give your patient a diphenhydramine injection to prevent complications. You should also shave the area around it and sharpie around the perimeter because these can shrink, so this helps you with margins at surgery if it changes size.

Initial treatment: Ok, so you diagnosed a mast cell tumor. Now what? To start, you want to ensure your patient is treated with medications in order to prevent complications that can occur secondary to degranulation. The dog will remain on these medications until you receive your biopsy back to determine if it was completely excised. What are these medications we speak of?

- **Pepcid (H2 blocker: famotidine)**: 1 mg/kg SID or ½ mg/kg BID. We prefer SID for ease of administration.

- **Prilosec (proton pump inhibitor: omeprazole)**: 1 mg/kg SID. While it might seem repetitive to do two gastroprotectants, a lot of research shows this drug works best. It is not easy to dose in small patients, so we just add it in with patients where the capsule size works. It is also available in liquid form at some human pharmacies.

- **Benadryl (H1 blocker: diphenhydramine)**: 2.2 mg/kg BID.

- **+/- Prednisone (steroid)**: 1mg/kg SID x 7 days, then decrease by 25% weekly until the histopathology results return after surgical removal or until recheck around 3-4 weeks (whichever comes first pending what your owner chooses to do). You do not always have to add this medication in, but some report an anti-cancer effect. Practically, we often use it for larger tumors that need to be made smaller for surgery, since it can be helpful at decreasing the size of the mass. Very small tumors may shrink up to where you cannot visualize them easily. Dr. Jeff wanted to mention that steroids are also highly recommended if clinical signs secondary to the MCT are present.

To recap, you have now diagnosed your patient with a mast cell tumor. You have no idea what grade it is because you can ONLY determine this through histopathology. How do you explain this to the owner, and what are your next steps doc?

Immediate client communication points:

1. First things first: For any mass, **let your owner know that there are benign and malignant causes** (The end – do not go down the rabbit hole of listing out ten types.). Let them know that the easiest way to gain further insight is through a needle sample and cytology. Many owners think you can tell them what the mass is from the exam, so explain that a needle sample is a very small sample and doesn't always give the full picture. It is a screening test and definitive diagnosis sometimes requires a bigger sample via biopsy/removal. If they're still not convinced, you can add that some masses can "play pretend" and be malignant resembling a benign fatty tumor like a lipoma.

    a. Explain that your needle sample and cytology is the least invasive way to gain more information without sedation and surgery. DO NOT FORGET to explain to owners that sometimes we DO NOT get an answer from cytology. Owners assume a test = definitive answers, but this is not always the case.

        i. **Communication tip from Dr. Jeff:** Avoid calling an FNA or "needle sample" a "needle biopsy." This can cause push back if a true biopsy is needed in the future by you or a referral clinician. I cannot tell you how many times I've heard "We already did a biopsy!" and it was just an FNA.

b. Discuss that there are many masses we can differentiate from in-house cytology, but there are some that require a pathologist at an outside lab for further review. A second opinion can be important if it means the diagnosis changes the plan and prognosis for their pet.

2. So now, you have your diagnosis. **This is where we LOVE handouts!** If your clinic does not have handouts, there are plenty of good resources online you can print. We use the Veterinary Partner website often. A good tip if you do not know how to have the conversation with an owner on a disease is to read the handout too. Oftentimes, these client handouts simplified our medical spiels and are a good way to learn lingo that is client friendly. Bring the handout in with you and show the owner a picture of the cytology (You can take a picture with your phone). Showing your client the results is a way to provide value to what you are doing, and they tend to be more amenable to cost when they can see the results too.

3. **Now, here is our example conversation once we have a diagnosis of MCT.**

   a. *"Mrs. Jones, so unfortunately, Petey's mass came back as a skin cancer called a mast cell tumor. I printed you a handout to review at home, but I want to go over a plan for this visit as well as our next steps. Mast cell tumors can spread to other areas of the body, as well as cause other changes due to the nature of the mass like vomiting, diarrhea, and stomach ulcers. I want to treat Petey with Benadryl right now so that we can prevent any complications from me manipulating the mass today with the sampling. It will be an injection I give him right now. Is that ok with you?"*

      i. Most owners are completely on board with this, and we let them know we are going to get the injection, while they start reading the handout.

   b. *"Now that we have given him the injection, let's talk about our plan moving forward. Unfortunately, I cannot tell how severe this mass is today. We have to do surgery to remove this mass completely, and then send it to the lab for further testing. This next test allows us to determine what grade it is because higher grades can be more likely to spread to other organs inside the body, while lower grade masses are curable with surgery if we are able to remove the mass completely. Surgery will be our next step, and I am happy to get you an estimate for it. I want to prepare you that oftentimes these incisions are very big because I want to make sure we get this mass off Petey to try to avoid a second surgery."*

c. You want to then discuss your estimate, basic surgical complications, and get the procedure scheduled. Make sure to also do blood work that day to ensure their dog is systemically healthy prior to anesthesia.
    i. There are many other tests that are recommended like x-rays, ultrasound, local lymph node aspirates, etc. It can get very expensive, so as a general practitioner, we find that the best first steps are cytology and blood work. Then, surgery. If histopathology shows that it is a lower grade, well differentiated tumor, then complete surgical excision is curative, and these have low risk of recurrence/spreading. If you find it is a higher grade, then you have more ammo to push for all these additional diagnostics to be thorough. This will be especially important if they want to see an oncologist after surgery.
    ii. Some owners will want to be proactive and do chest and abdominal x-rays prior to surgery. It is never wrong to at least offer x-rays as an easy test you can do if they want to be thorough, especially in an older patient (>7 years). You can offer to do them that day (have them drop off their pet) or plan to do them when their dog is sedated the day of surgery. We prefer to do x-rays the day of surgery to decrease stress on the patient and avoid getting behind on our busy appointment days. Dr. Jeff wanted to share that most specialists prefer abdominal ultrasound (over abdominal x-rays) if you have easy access to a referral center and the owner wants to be thorough. Traveling radiologists are also available in some cities that can be scheduled as well.
    iii. If they are cost conscious, the most important thing to do is to get the mass off and send it for histopathology. That way, you have at least removed the tumor and can get a grade to guide prognosis for that owner.

****ALWAYS send these tumors off for histopathology. Granted, some owners may be extremely financially limited, but it is SO helpful with prognosis and owner preparation. We have had masses come back as grade II (intermediate) and incompletely excised, despite an aggressive surgery. If we had known that, the owner would have been better prepared that it could regrow and potentially spread internally.** Prognosis is much poorer on the higher grade masses.

Dr. Jeff tip: Build your histopathology into the estimate. You do not have to present the histopathology as a separate "high-end/low-end" option but rather as a mandatory part of the package. If your owner has extreme financial concerns, this is the time to work with your manager or supervisor on adjustments (if your clinic allows). All efforts should be made to not cut corners on histopathology for this type of mass.

Surgical excision: This is always the treatment of choice. Try to get at least two cm margins around the mass and one fascial plane deep for the best chance of complete excision. Incompletely excised tumors often require a second surgery +/- radiation.

Prognosis: Grading, staging, and surgical excision are the main dictators of prognosis.

Grading a MCT

You may see multiple classification systems on your mast cell histopathology. The most commonly used systems are:

- Patnaik (3-tier) system with grades I, II, III. Grade III being the most malignant.
- Kiupel (2-tier) system indicates simply "low grade" or "high grade". "High grade" intuitively indicates more malignancy.

It is important to know they exist and the basics. In practice you will always be able to refresh yourself on the nuances of your individual case results with a book (or trusted academic website or scientific article) prior to calling the owner with results.

In general, lower grade tumors (such as grade I) are cured with complete surgical excision. Higher grade tumors that are incompletely excised have a poorer prognosis. Oftentimes grade II-III tumors, especially those that have spread to local lymph nodes, are of the poorest prognosis with median survival time ranging from three months to a year.

Best care is to offer referral to an oncologist for multi-modality therapy including chemotherapeutics and radiation.

- **Pro tip from Dr. Jeff:** If you do not have a local oncologist, touch base with the nearest internal medicine specialist. Some will also take on oncology cases depending on their residency training.

- Even if your client cannot afford referral, you can still call a local oncologist to discuss the case, as many are willing to consult with you. You can offer to the owner that they can at least go for the initial consult/exam fee to talk with an oncologist for further detail. They are not committed to treatment but rather will be able to get a good idea of what the different options cost, the side effects, etc. since many offer aggressive to palliative treatment plans. These consult fees have increased over the years, so make sure you know what your specialist charges in the area.
  - **Pro tip from Dr. Jeff:** It may also be good to remind them that most chemotherapeutics protocols are designed to make dogs have as little secondary illness as possible and they typically do not result in hair loss with the doses of medications utilized.

- Lastly, if they cannot afford referral and it is a higher grade MCT, you may be able to order Palladia (toceranib) or do the lowest-effective steroid dose for that patient long term. Anytime a part or all of a mast cell tumor remains on a patient, we will at minimum keep them on the oral medications mentioned earlier (famotidine, omeprazole, and diphenhydramine). For those that have more significant side effects or multiple tumors, prednisone can also be utilized. Sometimes, we will just add prednisone in for 3-4 week courses as needed when adverse clinical signs occur to minimize side effects of prednisone. The goal is to maintain a good quality of life while avoiding the adverse clinical signs of a MCT for as long as we can. Periodic bloodwork is also recommended with chemotherapeutics and long-term steroid use.

Final client communication points:

1. It is important to warn owners that even with complete excision of a lower grade tumor, new MCT can occur. They must ALWAYS monitor for new masses on their pet. We have had several patients continue to develop MCTs periodically. As long as they continue to be lower grades, we surgically remove them, and then continue to have parents monitor for new ones.

2. Make sure an owner understands that we should never ignore a mass on a patient that has had a mast cell tumor, as they can all look different. Performing cytology on every new mass as soon as they are noticed is the best way to be proactive in the future.

3. Not everyone can afford surgery, so we both have successfully medically managed these patients on oral medications when surgery is not an option. We have seen these patients live longer than we would expect on orals alone. Just warn the owner of all adverse signs that can occur and potential for poor, long-term prognosis.

Case example of recurrent MCT management

Dr. Gray's family dog, a 9 yr FS Golden Retriever

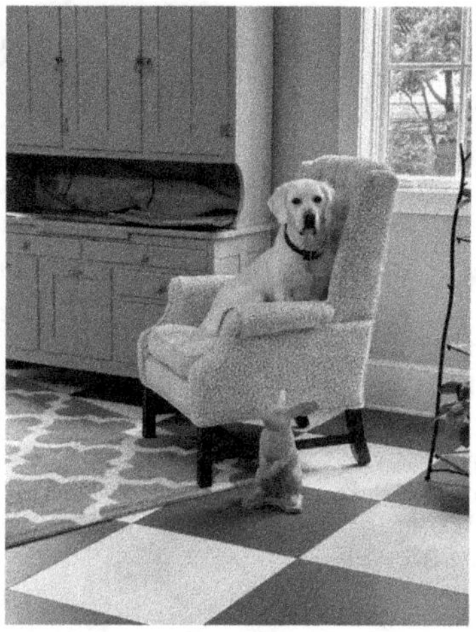

- As of 12/25, Stormy has had 9 MCTs removed. All have been low grade and completely excised. Their frequency has been one to a few popping up every 1-2 years roughly. One was on her tail and required her tail be docked to get good margins.
- My parents got pet insurance when she was a puppy, and they have had the majority of her medical bills covered ~90%: medications, treatments, diagnostics (doesn't cover exams or vaccines).
- **Here is how she has been managed medically by her GP and specialty team:**
  - Purina HA diet
  - I'm-Yunity mushroom supplement BID
  - Vetriscience Immune Support BID
  - Nordic Natural Algae Omega: BID
  - Benadryl 25 mg: 2 T PO BID
  - Famotidine PRN
  - Fortiflora probiotic SID
- **Here is how she has been managed with monitoring:**
  - Vet visits every 6 months to both her general practice vet and oncologist
  - Oncologist does majority of diagnostics: exam, blood work, chest x-rays, abdominal ultrasound

Non-surgical option to consider: Stelfonta! (*2025)

Stelfonta is an intratumoral injection being utilized by oncologists and GPs for MCTs of any grade that have not metastasized and are on areas surgically difficult to excise (example: distal limbs, face, ear). It could also be considered for a patient that is a high-risk anesthetic candidate. Stelfonta shares on their website that it destroys 87% of MCT within 1-2 injections. *See their website for a complete discussion guide.*

Virbac has a calculator to get your dosage based on tumor size. It is a single injection and then you inject in a fan pattern to get it throughout the tumor. ***It does sting a little so a way to minimize this is by allowing it to get to room temperature in the syringe prior to injection.*

Common side effects to share with your client include swelling, redness, bruising, pain and lameness. It is also important they understand the mass does necrose and fall off, leaving an open wound to heal by second intention within 4-6 weeks. A little over 50% of patients healed by day 28 and around 75% by day 42. It is recommended to recheck your patient every 7 days until healed.

In case you recheck a patient and do not have comfortability with this drug, it is important to remember that most dogs do NOT need antibiotics, e-collars or bandages to heal.

References:

- Muller, George H., et al. Muller & Kirk's Small Animal Dermatology. 7th ed., Elsevier, 2013.
- Welle, Monika M., et al. "Canine mast cell tumours: a review of the pathogenesis, clinical features, pathology and treatment." *Veterinary dermatology* vol. 19,6 (2008): 321-39. doi:10.1111/j.1365-3164.2008.00694.x
- Dobson J, Scase T. "Advances in the diagnosis and management of cutaneous mast cell tumours in dogs", J Sm An Prac. 2007. 48, 424–431DOI: 10.1111/j.1748-5827.2007.00366.x
- Brown, G., Finlay J., Straw R, et al. "Treatment of multiple synchronous canine mast cell tumours using intratumoural tigilanol tiglate", Front. Vet. Sci. 9 (2022)

NOTES:

NOTES:

Dental Disease

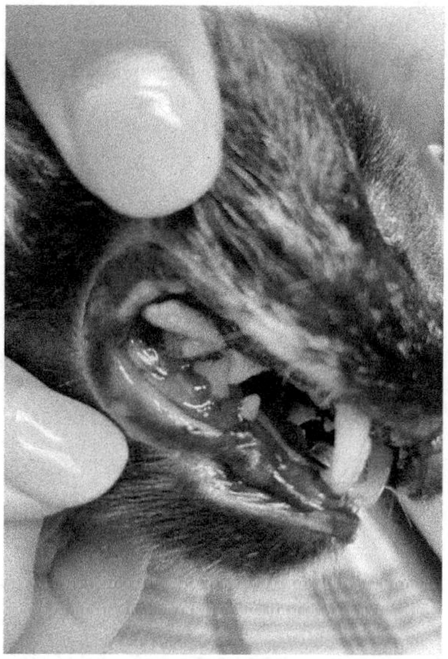

Dental disease will be one of THE most common diseases you diagnose in your patients. Dentistry is becoming one of the fastest areas of growth for companion animal practice. At least half of your patients will have some form of dental disease, and many practices are only treating 10% or less of these patients. WHY!? We feel that it comes down to a lack of training in vet school as well as a lack of equipment at some practices. It is too bad dental disease still only comprises ~0.1% of what you learn in vet school. If you feel less confident in this area, isn't it natural for you to shy away from it?

We both felt extremely self conscious with dentistry and did not know where to start when having this conversation with owners. You will find that a huge component of your wellness visits will be focused on this topic where you will discuss preventative care tips, dental cleaning procedures, and more. It can be a difficult topic to discuss because many owners are leary of anesthesia when it comes to a cleaning, or they have never even thought about brushing their pet's teeth. There is an art to how you communicate the importance of dentistry to owners. Many owners will get on board, while others will brush off your recommendations. So, how do you get compliance?

We are here to give you the skinny! Both of us started out with minimal training in dentistry and are now OBSESSED with it. It took us time, patience, and practice. We know that you can get there too.

It begins with the annual exam

Ok, let's start by getting you on the same page as your client. The majority of pet owners are not even aware of what is going on in their pet's mouth. Typically, owners only notice halitosis as a clinical sign because they are not even looking at their pet's premolars or molars. You will be amazed to find owners do not even realize their dog's teeth are covered in a "tartar retainer" until you show them.

Tip one: SHOW the owner what you are looking at, as you are discussing dental disease. You can either show them on their pet or take a photo for them to look at. Explain what these symptoms mean. What is gingivitis telling us? What is this tartar doing to their pet's teeth?

When your owner can visualize the problem, they are less likely to ignore it. Tip one goes a long way. You have to make the disease real for the owner and relating it to their own dental care will make many owners take it more seriously. So, now your owner is listening. What do you recommend the owner do for their pet?

Tip two: Use a grading scale and determine what grade of dental disease you are looking at. Many hospitals have a scale they use already. The most common is Grade 0-4. Tell the owner the grade and what it means.

- Grade 0: mild tartar accumulation, no gingivitis
- Grade 1: mild to moderate tartar present, gingivitis present
- Grade 2: moderate to severe tartar present, early periodontitis with <25% bone loss
- Grade 3: severe tartar present, established periodontitis with 25-50% bone loss
- Grade 4: severe tartar present, advanced periodontitis with >50% bone loss

Once you have your grade, you can determine the best course of action for your patient. Typically, grade 2-4 cannot be confirmed without dental x-rays. However, you can get a pretty good idea when you do your exam, and smell, your patient's oral cavity. Grade 0-1 often can be treated initially at home with your oral care recommendations. However, in grade 1 patients where the gingivitis is more diffuse, this would be an indication that a full dental cleaning is indicated. Grade 2-4 are times when a dental cleaning is strongly recommended, and it is important to warn an owner that there may be teeth that are infected. When you prep an owner early for tooth extraction risk, they are more willing to accept your recommendations when you call during the cleaning.

Tip three: Always provide an estimate that INCLUDES dental x-rays. It should NOT be elective because it is an important part of your oral exam. You will miss a lot of dental disease if you do not perform x-rays because many abscesses or resorptive lesions do not show disease above the gum line. When you offer services as a group estimate, they are less likely to say no.

Provide your owner with a complete estimate that covers anesthesia, monitoring, fluids, dental x-rays, scaling, polishing, fluoride, oral exam, and any other additives your clinic includes in a routine prophylactic cleaning. You can offer the estimate as a lump sum or range. We have found that owners respond better to a lump sum cost, saying it is around $500 for the procedure because they can grasp the cost better this way. If we are worried about infection or need for extraction, we tell the owner that the cost could go up as high as $1,000 if additional procedures are needed. If you word it this way, it allows the owner time to process the higher cost becauses it will depend on what is found while their pet is under anesthesia.

Never forget to explain the value of what this large number includes when discussing your estimate with your client. Owners need to know why this procedure is important in order for them to "buy in." You have all this knowledge from school to spill and can even relate it to human dentistry because many people value oral health.

Some tips include explaining how it prevents their pet from losing teeth over time, prevents and treats acute or chronic pain, how dental disease has links to heart and kidney disease if untreated, and more. The most effective strategies are when you explain that the goals of routine oral care, both at home and with anesthetic cleanings, are to prevent their pet from being in pain or losing teeth. The more routine we are, the less issues their pet has later on. Another important point to make is that this means their pet is not under anesthesia as long because we are preventing disease. The anesthetic risk increases the longer a patient is under anesthesia, so these routine short cleanings are easier on their pet, instead of having a four hour dental to extract 15 teeth (not to mention the pain!).

Tip four: Sure, this is a lot to discuss at a yearly appointment along with everything else, so we want to discuss ways to save time on this conversation. Come up with a quick spiel you give the owner while explaining the grade their pet is at as you show them their pet's dental disease. At the end of the appointment, you can plan to send them with a comprehensive estimate and some dates you are available to perform the procedure. You will be doing blood work on their pet that day to assess their health for anesthesia, so this gives you the perfect next time to call the owner and finalize the conversation. You can answer any last questions the owner has about the procedure, while you let the owner know their pet is healthy for anesthesia.

Let's talk through an example conversation

You: *"Mrs. Smith, as I am looking at Hugo's teeth, I am noticing that he has some bad breath, tartar build up, and redness along his gums. His breed is prone to dental disease. Have you noticed this?"*

Owner: *"Why no, I hadn't noticed."*

You: *"So, if you look here, these areas are where a large amount of tartar is stuck to his teeth. The longer this tartar stays here, the more risk Hugo is of losing teeth due to infection. He is at a grade 2/4 right now, so he will strongly benefit from a dental cleaning. Has your pet ever been through this before?"*

Owner: *"No, I have never gone through this before with a pet. Part of the reason why is I am nervous about anesthesia. I have heard pets can die under anesthesia, so it has always made me nervous the older my pet gets."*

You: *"I completely understand your concern, Mrs. Smith. There are some common misperceptions about anesthesia. As you know, there is always risk with anesthesia, whether you are a human or a dog. The risk for a healthy dog is extremely low, as it is a very controlled procedure. We monitor our patients very closely, can reverse or give medications if needed, and we provide them with fluids during the procedure that also help their body. The more routine we are with addressing his dental disease, the less time he is under anesthesia. My goal for today is to ensure Hugo is healthy for anesthesia, and we can also perform some lab work today to be thorough. If he appears healthy, his risk is very low for a complication."*

Owner: *"Ok, that all makes sense. Thank you for explaining it better to me. I certainly do not want my baby in pain and want the best for him."*

You: *"I completely understand. I will plan to send you with an estimate today, as well as our dental paperwork for you to review, so that you can prepare for the procedure. When I follow up with labwork results within the week, I am happy to answer any further questions you have for me."*

Tip five: Every yearly appointment should leave with some preventative care dental tips. You can print handouts that go over dental care tips or create your own. We make sure to mention to the owner a list of products we like to use that they can purchase with us or online.

A few brands we recommend are OraVet, Tartar Shield, and Maxi-Guard products. Use the Veterinary Oral Health Council for further information (www.vohc.org), as their seal is present on all approved dental care products.

Lastly, there are not many true dental emergencies. The two most common emergencies you will encounter are a tooth root abscess and a fractured tooth. Many times, you can start these patients on oral antibiotics (Clindamycin is the most common choice.) and a pain medication (Anti-inflammatory is a good choice.). Get them scheduled within 3-5 days, and these patients should be fine to wait until then.

If a tooth is mal-positioned and causing immediate pain, you can use injectable sedation and local blocks to remove it that day. Be sure to then schedule them for a follow up dental procedure within the week, as there may be other affected teeth. You can get full mouth x-rays and confirm the tooth was extracted completely. You will also be able to close the extraction site and be more thorough when the pet is under general anesthesia.

If you have a board-certified dentist in town, get to know them because you will have clients interested in referral. Learn what services they provide so you can offer these to your clients. Anytime you are performing a dental cleaning, make sure you know ahead of time if an owner would be interested in a root canal. Oftentimes, this is an option on your dental paperwork they sign to approve this procedure. Some owners are open to these advanced procedures, especially if it is a working dog, so you should know what your dentist charges for this procedure to prepare an owner.

How do you grow your dentistry skills?

- **Do an externship with a dentist or a general practice** that performs a lot of dentistry while you are in vet school. Consider shadowing a dentist after graduation if you have one local and want to learn more from a specialist.

- Do **online dentistry C.E. courses**.

- We strongly **recommend attending in person dentistry C.E. courses** after a few months out in practice. Many conferences or local dentists have lectures followed by wet labs where you work through feline and canine extractions on cadavers. You will already have some experience here, so the wet lab will make a lot more sense than when you were in vet school. These opportunities are great because you get to practice under a dentist and are able to improve your weaker areas.

- **Tell your colleagues you want practice**. Have them come get you when they have pathology on an x-ray so that you can practice reading x-rays. After you read the x-ray, examine the tooth so you can compare the x-ray findings to the oral exam. Tell them what you are thinking with your plan, so they can appropriately guide you.

- **PRACTICE!** Initially, you can shadow other veterinarians in your practice until you get comfortable. Make sure to talk through the steps with them so you know exactly what to do, as well as learn what instruments to use for each tooth (elevators, burrs, etc.). Ask if they have tips for extracting certain difficult teeth. Then, get started on your own dentals. You will always have someone nearby to help you if you have any issues. ALWAYS get in the habit of performing a post-extraction x-ray to ensure the roots were completely removed.

NOTES:

NOTES:

NOTES:

Diabetes Mellitus in Dogs

Reviewed by Dr. Jessica Romine, DVM, DACVIM

Nothing will slow your day down like a case of diabetes mellitus showing up on your schedule! We easily spent 2-3 hours on these appointments when we first started out and even now as there is a lot of information for owners to digest! Some clients will come to you with a suspicion of the disease, while others will have no idea. Let's discuss how you should approach these for optimal results.

Here is our basic approach to diabetes

Diagnosis:

1. CBC/Chemistry/Electrolytes and Urinalysis: the presence of **hyperglycemia and glucosuria together** is the **hallmark of diabetes**. Be sure to get both.

    a. UA: in addition to looking for glucosuria, **always screen for ketones in the urine of diabetics.** Presence of ketones → diabetic ketoacidosis. This makes treatment different compared to straightforward diabetes. Consider hospitalization in these patients, especially if they are systemically ill and anorexic.

    b. Fructosamine: consider adding on a fructosamine if you feel you need further confirmation (or if you are having difficulty making sense of your recent glucose curve). Occasionally, you will have a sick patient with blood glucose around the 300's and question the diagnosis.

    c. Dr. Jess Tip: Other things you might see commonly with new diabetics are...
        i. Pseudohyponatremia (analyzers will read quite low sodium because of the high glucose and high cholesterol)

ii. High total solids on the refractometer (triglycerides are solids too, so you'll get false readings)
iii. Potassium might seem okay...but if they are acidotic, it's falsely elevated and will drop with correction
iv. Look for creamy serum when separated - this means high triglycerides and is very common in diabetics. It may need treatment to reduce chances of pancreatitis!

2. Urine culture: in addition to a urinalysis, a urine culture should be performed at time of diagnosis and periodically throughout the management of diabetes if finances allow. As you know, diabetics are also prone to secondary complications such as pancreatitis, urinary tract infections, etc.

Talking points to owners:

1. **Give an overview of the disease process**. Start your discussion on the general concept of managing diabetes. Here is an example conversation.

   - *"Fluffy has been diagnosed with diabetes, which is a metabolic disease where her body no longer produces insulin. In dogs, this is Type 1 diabetes, which means the pancreas has stopped making insulin completely. It's important to understand that, unlike Type 2 diabetes in people, this can't be reversed or corrected with weight loss or changes in diet alone, even though those things will still play a very important role in managing her condition. Because her body can't make insulin, Fluffy will need insulin injections for the rest of her life in order to survive. Without insulin, her blood sugar levels will remain dangerously high, which can make her feel very unwell and lead to serious, potentially life-threatening complications. But with the right treatment and support, many dogs with diabetes go on to live happy, good-quality lives."*

     - Now take a deep breath. Ask if the owner has any familiarity with the disease (many people have family members with it). You will want to assess if your client seems to understand, so that you have permission to keep talking.

   - *"As a diabetic, she will now need injections of insulin with her meals twice a day. The good news is that insulin needles are really small and most pets do not even know they are getting an injection."*

 - ▽ We like to bring in a syringe for the owner to see what it looks like because many people are scared of this part. Once the owner sees that the insulin needle is small, they often feel better.

2. **Goals of treatment:** We always set up the expectation from the beginning that diabetes *can* be difficult to manage. Most regulate well, but some you will have trouble with regulating early on. Our goal is NOT to maintain blood sugar close to normal at all times (which is what they do for humans), but rather to improve clinical signs (maintain weight, decrease thirst and urination to a manageable state, and prevent secondary complications from occurring such as urinary tract infections, pancreatitis, etc.).

   - ▶ Tip from Dr. Jess: You should really emphasize this point because a lot of people get overwhelmed by the diagnosis and treatment. There is a lot more flexibility in animals in how we control them because we are not worried about heart attacks, kidney damage, wound problems, etc. that people get with long-term diabetes. I usually say if my patients live most of their lives in the 150-300 range, that's amazing because it's probably below the PU/PD threshold but above the hypoglycemia risk threshold.

3. **Food choice and food timing with insulin:** Explain that with diabetics, insulin is to be given with food at a set time that is every 12 hours (7 am and 7 pm for example). If the owner is ever off by an hour, no big deal, but just let them know that most of the time they need to be consistent.

   - ▶ Twice a day feedings only. No treats or snacks in between, as this can cause an unwanted blood sugar spike. This can be really hard for owners, but you have to explain how it impacts the treatment. If an owner wants to give a treat, such as a dental chew, we will tell them to give it shortly after meal time when the insulin is kicking in.
     - ▽ If they are struggling with this point, Dr. Jess recommends sharing this: Even if their dog is hungry, giving food without insulin (like a midday snack) won't help because without insulin the glucose can't go into their cells. All they're doing is spiking their dog's blood sugar. Commiserate with them!

   - ▶ We find that for most owners the easiest way is to give the injection *while* the pet is eating.

4. **Insulin and syringe choice:** Generally, we use an intermediate acting insulin such as Vetsulin (insulin of choice, but it can be cost prohibitive for large dogs or some clients) or Humulin-N/ Novolin-N (more affordable, have owner's look up which is cheaper - GoodRx.com is a great website you can recommend). Just be sure to warn an owner that the human insulin types can make regulation difficult. Dr. Jess's insulin of choice as of 2026 is Toujeo, but it is more expensive than the other options. Feel free to look into it further if interested.

    - We make our choice based on the owner and the financial situation. Explain both insulin types and that the difference is in the way they are formulated. The generic ones at Walmart are better suited to humans. If they choose the generic brands, you must let them know that if we cannot regulate their pet well on this type, we may have to go to a more expensive option. The human generic options can sometimes make regulation more difficult, or require more glucose curves to find the right amount.

    - Whenever it makes sense, **ALWAYS impress on the client how powerful insulin is as a molecule.** Even just making small changes on their own can have a big impact on their pet (and where hypoglycemia is concerned, even death). Because of this, it is important to give it as directed and never change the dose without consulting you first.

    - U-40's vs U-100's. Let the owner know that each type of insulin has a special syringe that must go with it. If they use the wrong type, their dog could face life threatening consequences due to the change in dose. On your insulin Rx, always write: only give with U-40 (Vetsulin) syringes or only give with U-100 (Novolin-N) syringes.

5. **Insulin administration and storage:** It is great to teach a tech how to explain this part to save you time. We always let the owner know that this information is located on the pamphlet that is in each bottle, so they can read through it at home.

    - There are two ways to prep the bottle: Humulin-N or Novolin-N need to be rolled, whereas Vetsulin needs to be shaken in order to get the medication mixed together properly. Offer Vetsulin pens for owners who might be concerned with correct dosing, especially in small animals where pulling up a few units can be tricky (example: elderly clients may be a good candidate for pens). Make sure your client understands how to prime the pen first before every injection and show them if possible. *Your client can always schedule a recheck visit once they have the drug to do together to help them practice.*

- Bring in an insulin syringe and show the owner how to measure it because insulin syringes are TINY and often do not have numbers next to every line. **This is one place you do not want owners to get confused.** Have them practice drawing up sterile saline, and then have them administer this to their pet for practice. Owners feel much more confident once they have practiced with you.

- Remember to tell owners they need to rotate sides of the pet, and location, regularly. If they give the injection in the same spot every time, this can decrease its efficacy later due to scar tissue formation.

6. **Follow-up plan:** Let them know that we will start with a blood glucose curve in 1 week to assess response to therapy. We continue to perform curves until we find the right dosage for their pet. Warn them that it can sometimes take 2-3 dose adjustments requiring multiple curves. Dr. Jess recommends that you really stress these rechecks and keep them weekly until controlled because the longer it takes to get the dog controlled, the more frustrated the owner will become. You will almost always be increasing the dose at least once.

    - Once regulated, we plan on seeing their pet every 6 months for routine lab-work (CBC, chemistry, UA, T4) in order to keep up with their health. If they are well controlled and clinically doing well, we usually recommend a blood glucose curve 2 times a year.

    - If a client cannot afford frequent routine testing, use clinical signs such as assessment of PU/PD, energy, appetite, etc. to guide you and see if you can negotiate at least one glucose curve a year and one bloodwork and urinalysis. Warn the client about what we may miss by not being thorough, but you need to prioritize testing for your clients that are financially limited.

    - **Glucose curves:** There are three options, and **we always recommend starting with in-clinic glucose curves or Freestyle Libre curves (which are always inserted and calibrated in the clinic)** until the patient is well regulated.

        - **Three options:**

            - **In-clinic blood glucose checks** as a drop off for the day were recommended commonly until new technology gave us a better option. Reasons why include it often doesn't reflect a dog's normal day/routine, the results are influenced by stress and hospitalization, and they are the same cost as a Libre. Dr. Jess states that she almost exclusively does Freestyle Libre curves now.

- **Freestyle Libre®**: This is a continuous glucose monitoring system you place on your patient which monitors glucose via the interstitial fluid. It lasts about 10-14 days and has a sensor and reader component. The reader can be reused in the future, but they must get a new sensor each time you want to reapply the libre. You have to calibrate the sensor and reader in the hospital first with some readings, so be sure to find an appropriate online resource to guide you on this process. The benefit to this method is most animals tolerate it very well and if owners scan as directed while at home, you can get a better idea of regulation without the stress of 'pricks' at the hospital.
    - **Here is how Dr. Jess does it:** We charge a cost for applying the Libre. The owner can buy it from the hospital or get it with a prescription from a pharmacy for us to apply once it has been picked up. We use tissue glue to keep it adhered. We then have a daily interpretation cost that they pay. Typically we tell owners we look about 4 times through the curve unless there are issues, or you can just charge a flat fee. It works out the same as all those in-house BG collections and much less stressful for their pet.

- **AlphaTrak® at home**: Owners can be taught **to perform the curve at home**. They must buy the AlphaTrak®, and we do not generally offer this until after the initial curve or two.
    - Remind owners who do curves at home to always report them to you and never change insulin on their own without consulting you first.

A few more Libre tips from Dr. Jess:

1. You don't have to calibrate it in house. It is applied, wait 1 hour, and then you can start reading it. You need a smartphone now, as I don't think you can get the readers anymore. A way around it for elderly is that you can add as many people as you want, so multiple family members (and hospital team members) can scan the same device. You can also set up a hospital LibreLink account online for free and give owners your practice ID to link via the LibreView app, and then you can see their data without having to get it from them.

2. It's definitely much preferred to see things day to day and you can be a lot more aggressive with dose increasing (i.e. go up daily until you're seeing the nadir below, say 300, and then wait a day or two, then keep increasing until you see a curve appear).

3. Do coach owners not to overinterpret the data, especially if it reads low. The monitor is accurate within about 20-40 units, so if it says "low, 45" it could be low, but it could also be totally normal at 75. Coach them to look at the dog clinically (mentation, energy, etc.) before determining if they need to intervene or not. See if they seem fine vs. if they are weak/lethargic/ADR before feeding a snack to increase blood sugar, as that will otherwise just mess them up with high glucose. Remember that it takes 15 minutes for interventions to show up on the curve, so if you do feed, wait 15 minutes before rechecking.

- ▽ Many owners are overwhelmed at this point, and so often we start by recommending one or two ways to do the glucose curve depending on overwhelm and briefly mention we can consider some other methods in the future. Ultimately, we want options that decrease stress for the patients and the owners to help with compliance. If choosing in-clinic curves, you want to make sure they stick to the same insulin routine the day of their drop off appointment. Clarify that they need to feed their dog when they give the insulin because many clients get confused by this. The owner should either drop their dog off first thing in the morning for your staff to do it or right after their morning meal/insulin dose (our preferred) if it allows for a reasonable monitoring period. Prep owners that their pet will be at the hospital all day (typically 10-12 hours based on how late your clinic is open).

- ▽ If your client wants to perform the curve at home (only for trusted owners/advanced users), have them purchase the Freestyle Libre (they will need a prescription for this) or they can purchase the AlphaTrak® glucometer online if they feel their pet will tolerate ear and paw pad pricks for readings. If your client does perform the curve at home, they must be trained so that they can get appropriate readings and then email you the results for interpretation.

4. **Short and long term expectations:**

- **Diabetics are prone to being ill, so close monitoring is important:** It is important to stress to owners that their pet is now immunocompromised and prone to becoming ill suddenly. This means that owners will always have to watch them closely for any signs of illness and alert you right away if they see them. Explain that pets with diabetes do not bounce back as quickly as they did previously, hence the importance of being so vigilant and communicating with you. Two serious complications we always bring up are hypoglycemia and diabetic ketoacidosis. With hypoglycemia, discuss that it can cause death and bring up the need for karo syrup in the home. With DKA, we briefly describe it as an illness that requires extensive hospitalization to get stabilized and feeling better.

- **Regulation can be difficult early on or later in the disease:** Set the expectation that most dogs with diabetes can live a good, long life once we get them regulated. Some dogs are outliers and challenging to get regulated from the start. Others will have challenges regulating later on in the disease. This is especially true when another disease is present elsewhere (such as Cushing's disease, cancer, etc.).

- **Diabetes is an expensive disease to manage.** Insulin, periodic glucose curves, food, and blood work/urine checks are all parts of the cost.

- **Quality of life:** Even though it is a difficult decision, it is fair to discuss humane euthanasia if the owner does not feel they can care for their pet with diabetes.

Client communication summary for diabetes mellitus in dogs

1. Overview of the disease
2. Goals of treatment
3. Food choice and food timing with insulin
4. Insulin and syringe choice
5. Insulin administration and storage
6. Follow-up plan
7. Short and long term expectations

Communication points we have forgotten that got us in trouble

- **Discussing cost of therapy:** Insulin can be very pricey. Many owners may say yes to treatment initially out of shock, but once reality sets in, they may not be able to afford it. You will want to give them a rough cost of insulin. You can tell them what it costs at your clinic versus the Goodrx website to compare insulin prices at nearby pharmacies. It is a cost factor to consider along with the cost of glucose curves and routine visits. Novolin-N is usually around $40-60 at this time in 2026.

- **Expectations while regulating:** Ensure your client that the Freestyle Libre monitoring route will improve speed to control, identification of problems, and compliance. It's much easier for them because they don't have to keep bringing in their dog, and their dog will have a lower stress level as well as not require frequent blood drawing at the hospital.
    - **We used to do this:** Prep them from the start that you will see a lot of each other initially, while you are figuring out the right dosage for their pet. Often, it takes between 2-4 curves, and we do these every 2-3 weeks after insulin adjustments. If you do not prep them for this, they can get frustrated with all the visits up front. By making them aware of this from the beginning, it sets up their expectations appropriately. *How tough on all involved, huh!? We love new technology and options to make things low stress for our patients and clients.*

- **Explain that things can get complicated with diabetes:** Discuss with owners that if we have trouble regulating their pet, it may mean we need to re-evaluate a few things. This can include how insulin administration is going at home or diagnostics to look for an infection (ear infection, urinary tract infection, pancreatitis, etc.). Even an ear infection can throw their curve off. If we do not find an obvious infection, consider imaging such as an abdominal ultrasound. Dr. Tarantino had a diabetic cat she could not get regulated that ended up having a pancreatic mass that was discovered on ultrasound. By performing an abdominal ultrasound, they were able to find the mass and understand why regulation was going poorly.

- **Nearly EVERY diabetic dog will develop cataracts:** Say this to the owner the first day! We both have had upset owners call because their pet became suddenly blind, and no one warned them about this complication.

    - You can say... *"Whether your dog's diabetes is controlled or not, cataracts will form over time causing your pet to become blind. The latest statistic as of 2025 was that about 85% of dogs would develop cataracts. The better regulated we keep your pet, the longer it takes for them to develop, as they can develop suddenly overnight to slowly over years. There is a surgery we can consider to remove them in the future that will restore your pet's vision."*

    - It is great to start dogs with cataracts on twice daily Flurbiprofen (anti-inflammatory eye drop) to decrease inflammation. Cataracts cause inflammation, and a lot of ocular diseases can occur secondary to cataracts.

- **Failing to tell them (and scare them a little) about how powerful insulin is:** We both learned the hard way that some people like to play doctor and try to avoid visits by adjusting insulin themselves. This is a dangerous game. Explain to your owners that insulin is a powerful molecule. They should NEVER adjust it themselves, as it is important we adjust things slowly based on blood glucose curves and doctor input. Discuss the risks of low blood sugar, so they understand how severe this can get. Explain the clinical signs of hypoglycemia so they can monitor for this complication, and recommend they keep some form of sugary syrup (karo syrup for example) on hand. That way, they can give it at home if the signs develop, and then call the hospital. Inform the owner that we err on the side of caution with insulin because hypoglycemia is always more dangerous than hyperglycemia.

- **Show them the exact mark on the insulin syringe for the dosage:** People get really confused about the dosage, so it is important to show them first. Then, let them show you, so you can see that they know the exact amount to administer. We have had people overdose and underdose sick dogs because the dose was being done incorrectly, so make a very big deal over this.

- **Discuss what to do if their pet will not eat:** This could be one of the first signs that their pet is ill. We always let them know that if their pet does not eat or eats only a small part of their meal, they should only give a HALF DOSE, and then call us. Based on how the pet is acting, the client may need to bring their pet in to be seen to determine why they are off their food.
    - **Tip from Dr. Jess:** I often arm my owners with anti-nausea and appetite stimulation medications to have on hand if they need them, so they can give a trial and see if they eat and can get all their insulin. Plus, if they still won't eat after that or vomit again, it confirms they definitely need to be seen by a vet.

- **Discussion on how long they can keep an insulin vial:** The pharmacy will label a vial to be good for only 30 days due to human health regulations. In Plumb's and in the veterinary literature, insulin can technically last longer. Most state 4-6 months if stored and managed appropriately. You must warn an owner though that efficacy could decrease the longer they have the bottle, which can impact their pet's regulation.

    - If regulation becomes poor suddenly, always be sure to ask this question about their insulin bottle. Sometimes, dogs will present with hypoglycemia due to a new vial being used after 4-6 months on the last vial or you can see the opposite where towards the end of the vial it is more potent because it wasn't being suspended well enough before doses.

Things to evaluate if you are having difficulty regulating a dog

- Ask these history questions to the owner:
  - Is the owner giving insulin appropriately?
  - Is the bottle too old?
  - Are they rolling or shaking?
  - Are they measuring to the appropriate level?
  - Are they feeding their pet outside of the regular schedule?
  - Are they on an appropriate food?
  - Did they change food recently?
  - Is someone in the household giving their dog treats outside of meal times?
  - Are they giving insulin in the same place?
  - Are they giving insulin at the same time of day?
- Any concurrent infections present? Ears? Urinary tract infection (i.e. perform a UA +/- urine culture).
- Consider a fructosamine. This test is falling by the wayside.
  - **Dr. Jess perspective on "How are you using this test in practice?":** I don't really use fructosamine often. As a diagnostic, I use it if we are trying to tell stress hyperglycemia from emerging diabetes (but if there is PU/PD, weight loss, etc I pretty much already have my answer. It is really for patients where the owner has not noticed anything. Dogs don't mount nearly as much of a stress hyperglycemia, so if there is any significant hyperglycemia it is diabetes in all likelihood. Similarly, Freestyle Libre monitoring has essentially taken over fructosamine in terms of monitoring for diabetic control. We will put a monitor on once or twice a year or if the owner is concerned it is not well-controlled and just see how things are going.
- Is a somogyi effect occurring?
  - **Interesting tidbit from Dr. Jess:** Somogyi effect is kind of a myth! It's probably actually the Dawn Phenomenon not working:
    - https://www.vin.com/apputil/content/defaultadv1.aspx?pId=20539&catId=113455&id=8506497&ind=344&objTypeID=17
- Is it time for imaging?
- Is there insulin resistance? (Consider if you are > 2.2 U/kg dose.)
- Other endocrinopathy or disease present? (CBC/chem/lytes/T4, abdominal ultrasound, etc.)

NOTES:

NOTES:

Diarrhea in Kittens

Reviewed by Dr. Jessica Romine, DVM, DACVIM

Common differentials for diarrhea in a kitten

- Dietary
- Infectious: bacterial, viral (panleukopenia, etc.), etc.
- Parasitic: giardia, coccidia, hookworms, roundworms, crypto, tritrichomonas, etc.
- Toxin
- Something else on DAMNIT-V that is not straightforward

Straightforward kitten diarrhea: Sounds simple right? Probably just worms...but then, why is the owner still calling you two days later complaining that nothing has changed or that symptoms are worsening? Here is our straightforward plan for kitten diarrhea in a stable, otherwise healthy kitten.

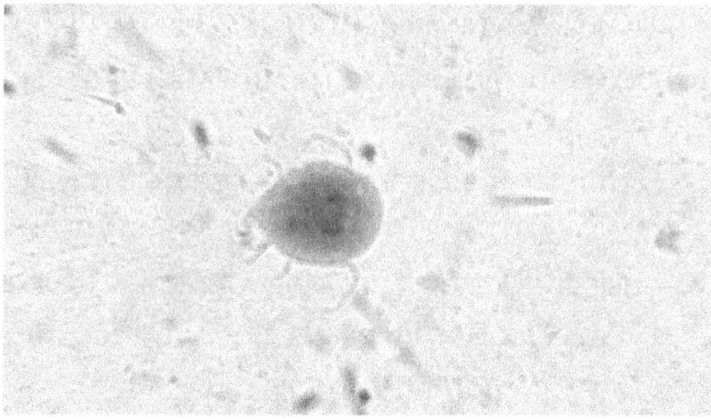

You can take our treatment plan step-by-step based on your physical exam, as you may not need all treatments initially.

Diagnostics: Be sure you know where this kitten came from with a good history. A shelter, a breeder, the streets, etc. will help you prioritize what this kitten has probably been exposed to, vaccinated for, dewormed against, diet exposure, etc. These are some of the tests we run to gain further information at the first to second visit.

- Fecal float, cytology, and direct smear
    - It is important to tell owners that fecal testing can help us to find a cause, but a negative fecal does not necessarily rule out parasites due to their life cycle and intermittent shedding.
- FIV/Felv combo test (if >2 lbs)
- Canine parvo test IF you are suspicious of panleukopenia based on clinical signs
- IFA/PCR fecal testing (to look for rarer differentials like crypto or tritrichomonas)
- Blood work such as a CBC and chemistry (can help to screen for organ dysfunction, secondary complications, or raise suspicion of a severe infection)

Treatment plan: Go step by step through your treatment plan. Oftentimes, we use severity to guide us in our choices. Many kittens with mild diarrhea at a first visit will respond well to a single dose of strongid, a probiotic, and a bland diet. These options will give you wiggle room to add on therapies based on their kitten's response to treatment along the way.

1. Strongid once, Panacur course for 3 days (liquid or powder formulation), +/- Albon.
2. Insist the kitten start a bland diet like Feline I/D for 2 straight weeks.
    a. Dr. Jess loves her fiber and recommends adding in a small amount of rice bran cereal to the food
3. Probiotic daily. Purina Fortiflora is an easy option for them to administer. See chronic diarrhea chapter for more options.
4. +/- Vitamin B12 injections. We usually do vitamin B12 0.1 mL SQ in kittens. Check dosing.

Client communication: Communicating that these cases can be frustrating up front is really important to get owners on the same page as you. This helps you switch plans as needed depending on diagnostics and the response to treatment.

Kitten diarrhea client communication summary

- Set the stage letting owners know it can be frustrating.
- Deliver your initial plan.
- Deliver your back up plan.
- Caution owners that if they worsen at any point, they need to call or come in.
- Reiterate plan or lay out next steps for owners that may need the extra assurance.

- **Set the stage:**
  - *"Kitten diarrhea can be frustrating and occur due to a variety of causes. The most common causes we see are due to parasites and diet, although I have seen a whole range of causes."*
- **Deliver your plan:**
  - *"Here is the plan I would like to put in place. We will first take a straightforward approach with a dewormer, probiotic, and a special bland diet I have here called I/D. I would like for you to call and give us an update in 2 days if your kitten is not improving. If there is no improvement in 2 days, I may add in additional medications like Albon for a parasite that may not be showing up on the fecal at this time or some fiber to the diet. Now, I do not anticipate the diarrhea to be 100% back to normal, but my hope is that it is getting more and more formed each day."*
- **Deliver your back-up plan:**
  - *"Now, if the diarrhea still persists after several days of starting the next treatment, I will need to see Ralph back for a recheck, as it is likely we will need to reassess and consider more testing or different treatments. That is where the diagnosis may get more complicated, but many of my patients respond well to my first treatment plan."*

- **Your caution:**
    - *"If at any point Ralph becomes more sick with worsening or new clinical signs, I need you to call us because this may mean something more serious is going on."*
- **If the owner still seems confused or overly concerned, you can drive it home one more time, but do not do this if you feel like they get it:**
    - *"I want to emphasize this again. Many kittens have a straightforward cause and resolve quickly with the plan I laid out, but sometimes kitten diarrhea requires extensive diagnostics. We are going to start with this plan to cover the most common causes first to see how your kitten responds before we dig deeper with further testing."*
- **Lastly, for owners that are really concerned, or you feel like they may blame you if something was not done or offered:** We will lay out the plan, and then discuss additional diagnostics that can be performed such as blood-work or a parvo test.
    - *"Your kitten appears stable today, but the goal of this testing at the first visit is to be thorough if you want to rule in/out a variety of causes."*
    - Usually, they will tell us no, so make sure to document what tests they declined. This approach allows you to be thorough and gives the client some room to decide what testing they want performed that day on their stable kitten.
    - By talking through the tests early on and what you will rule in/out, you are setting the foundation for a future visit if it is needed. Your client is prepared for diagnostics when their kitten's diarrhea is not resolving, and it makes it easier to get a 'yes' at the recheck. People respond well when they can see there is a path forward and a plan to follow.
        - Put a call back in for 24-48 hours to have your nursing team check in. If the kitten is not improving, have an estimate ready to send to your client so they can prepare ahead of time. We found this little trick helped us have smoother rechecks because we have a prepared client arriving for the appointment.

NOTES:

NOTES:

Flea Allergy Dermatitis in Cats

Reviewed by Dr. Jeff Tinsley, DVM, DACVD

We agree that this may seem like a simple topic, but just wait until you get multiple calls from frustrated owners because they STILL see fleas despite your best recommendations. It is a common client complaint and something you can easily prevent with the right talking points. Practicing in the south, fleas are our NEMESIS! We feel for the kitties (and dogs, of course) who battle flea allergies.

The biggest thing to remember when any household has a flea infestation is to first **ask how many other pets are in the household**. Time and time again, the reason a dog or cat is unable to get better is due to the owner not protecting all the pets in the household. We agree that this sounds like common sense, but many owners do not realize the life cycle of the flea. They also think that the only pet bothered by fleas in the household is the one with the hair loss, excoriations, and intense pruritus. Flea allergy dermatitis will not be seen with every pet that has fleas. Unaffected pets can act as carriers. It is only on those with a true allergy to flea saliva, and the intense pruritus that leads to all the secondary changes to the coat and skin that worry an owner enough to bring their cat in to be seen.

Rule #1: Explain to the owner that fleas actually bite their pet and take a blood meal. This freaks them out, and 9 times out of 10 they will get on board with parasite prevention. Then, they will better understand that this bite causes pruritus and the secondary changes that show their cat is very uncomfortable.

Rule #2: Go over the flea life cycle you spent so much time learning in parasitology. See... your classes did come in handy! They need to understand that adult fleas are only 5% of the population, so they are not seeing 95% of the infestation in their house!! Many cases in-clinic exhibit alopecia of the hind limbs and dorsal lumbosacral areas. These are hallmark areas seen in flea allergy dermatitis due to overgrooming from flea bites. During your exam, you should also comb the pet with a flea comb **with the client present**. This is often the best way to show an owner their cat has fleas.

Some tips to help you find fleas

1. If only flea dirt is seen, the comb will catch this too. If you place flea dirt on a paper towel and apply a small amount of water, rub the material then a light brown, red color may indicate that this flea poop was indeed a blood meal!

2. A fecal test that is positive for tapeworms may also indicate fleas were ingested from overgrooming. Anecdotally, some clinicians have identified tape worms from taping the rectum of cats and assessing for eggs under the microscope as well.

Rule #3: Discuss EXACTLY how the products work to break up the flea life cycle, and recommend products for all pets in the household. We always recommend every pet be protected year round. Many owners of indoor cats are skeptical of this, so it helps to explain to owners how we can bring fleas in on our clothes. We can be carriers too! You can also mention how mosquitos get in the house, and how many parasites that get in the house carry intestinal parasites. This explanation usually gets many owners on board with parasite prevention. It helps to come up with a spiel, so they understand there is still risk with an indoor only cat.

- Side note: We will not get too in depth with products here because there are so many. However, a **good tip for you** when you start your first job is to make sure you know what products your hospital carries before you start working. It makes it so much easier to recommend products when you can brush up on what each covers, how long they last, and how they work before you even start working. This extra step allows you to recommend the right product for each scenario you see.

- There are many products out there, and topical monthly Revolution Plus (selamectin + the isoxazoline: sarolaner) and Nexgard Combo (esafoxolaner, eprinomectin, and praziquantel) will always be crowd favorites due to their broad spectrum coverage for cats. An isoxazoline should also treat for itchy ectoparasites like feline scabies or Demodex gatoi (one of the few itchy species of Demodex). In fact, monthly products are preferred for true flea allergy cases when possible. However, if an owner has multiple pets or seems like they are struggling to grasp the concept of flea prevention, using a longer acting product like the topical Bravecto (fluralaner, lasts three months) or a Seresto collar (flumethrin and imidacloprid, lasts eight months) is reasonable. It can take two to three months to eliminate an infestation, and if they are delinquent in applying a monthly product, it will be even more difficult. The longer acting product may eliminate the infestation more effectively if there is poor compliance.

Rule #4: It is important to explain to owners that as long as their pet is protected AND appropriate deep cleaning is performed, the flea infestation will be eliminated. Even if they see adult fleas jump on and off their pet over the next month or so, it is a transient thing if they stay on top of your recommendations. It is **vital** that you discuss environmental deep cleaning measures with them like vacuuming (immediately getting rid of the bag), washing all bedding, etc. This is to remove all life cycles of the flea from the environment as they are extremely prolific at reproducing. In addition, some life stages survive for long periods in the carpet, cracks of hard wood floors, sofa, beds, etc until they are physically removed. Some resources recommend deep cleaning every 2 weeks for a minimum of 3 cycles to eliminate flea infestations. Outdoor treatments may be needed in especially high flea endemic areas.

Pro-Tip from Dr. Jeff

There are great client handouts online you can print and send home to save you time in the exam room too. I recommend https://veterinarypartner.vin.com which has several flea control handouts. As of this publication, they do not require a membership for most of their handouts. You can utilize your technicians to assist with flea education as well.

Rule #5: Lastly, if you are suspicious of flea allergy dermatitis beyond just a flea infestation, then it is important to perform skin cytology to identify and treat secondary bacterial (or yeast) infection on the skin along with pruritus.

- **Clinical signs may include:** flea dirt, pruritus, alopecia in the dorsal lumbosacral and/or hind limb areas, miliary dermatitis, eosinophilic granuloma complex and others may be seen.

- If bacterial infection is confirmed via skin cytology you can consider Convenia (cefovecin) the 2 week antibiotic injection as an empirical choice (if there have been no recent antibiotics). Unless the pyoderma is extremely minor, repeating this injection in 2 weeks for a full 4 week treatment is recommended.
- You can treat pruritus with a steroid such as a tapering dose of prednisolone . Cats can receive 1-2 mg/kg PO SID with a taper of roughly 25% per week until recheck at the 4 week recheck visit. Some clinicians decrease the dose every 5 days and/or go to every other day at the end of their tapers. Use your clinical judgement based on severity of the patient to determine your taper preference for each case.. Cats can do well with pills in Pill Pockets/Pill Wrap or mixed into wet food. You can also get pills compounded into a flavored liquid if necessary. Ask your technician to show owners how to medicate, so they will feel more confident when they go home. There are also great Youtube videos you can email to owners on feline medicating as well.
  - Some doctors will give a systemic steroid injections like Depomedrol (methylprednisolone), but there can be increased side effects with it and you have less control on dosing once it has been administered (vs. orals that can be discontinued immediately). This drug should last anywhere from 4-6 weeks in a cat. It should be reserved for cases where clients have failed orally medicating, despite

good veterinary guidance. In addition, if your steroids do not seem to last long enough, be sure to investigate concurrent differentials perpetuating the pruritus. *It is imperative you discuss possible risks to their cat such as the potential for developing conditions like diabetes, heart failure, etc., as we have seen this happen to some cats following a Depo injection.*

- Rechecking at the 4 week mark to assess for resolution of infection, status of pruritus and progress of deep cleaning compliance is also advised.

- Topical antimicrobials as adjunctive therapy are encouraged, like Miconahex Triz Mousse, but many cats are not a huge fan of products on their skin. Also, don't forget that *some* cats will allow medicated bathing for dedicated owners who want to reduce systemic antimicrobial use.

References:

- Muller, George H., et al. Muller & Kirk's Small Animal Dermatology. 7th ed., Elsevier, 2013.
- Mueller, R.S., Nuttall, T., Prost, C., Schulz, B. and Bizikova, P. (2021), Treatment of the feline atopic syndrome – a systematic review. Vet Dermatol, 32: 43-e8. https://doi.org/10.1111/vde.12933

NOTES:

NOTES:

NOTES:

Foreign Bodies in Dogs

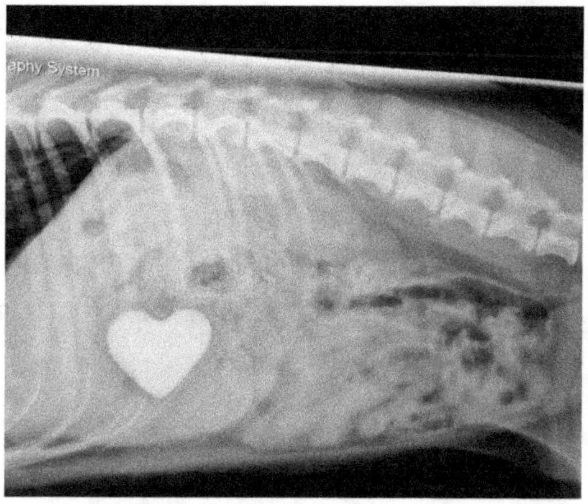

Acute vomiting in dogs will be a common sick appointment you see in general practice. While this symptom has a long differential list, foreign body ingestion will rank high in many of your cases. Think a young dog or certain stereotypical large breeds like a Labrador Retriever. When a foreign body is on the top of your differential list, you will find that it is not as black and white as you would like it to be. This diagnosis can be very frustrating and one of your more difficult cases as a new grad. Sometimes, you get lucky with a slam dunk corn cob staring you in the face on an x-ray (or that cute heart shaped paper weight in the x-ray above), but many times it will not be that clear cut. Obstruction cases present in many ways, and x-rays will be even more variable. Owners get easily frustrated when a veterinarian does not have an up front answer for them, and obstruction cases can commonly lead to client complaints if you are not careful. These cases really come down to communication, and we are here to help you navigate these difficult cases with ease.

Think of it this way. You have a two year old male neutered Labradoodle who presents for acute vomiting of two days duration. He has vomited seven times today and has not been able to hold down any food or water. He has not had any interest in food the last few days, and the owner has no idea what is causing these symptoms. The owner cannot confirm that a toy is missing or that he got into the trash. As an astute veterinarian, you know this case will benefit from x-rays, as the best diagnostic choice to guide you. You give the owner an estimate of $450, which includes your exam, x-rays, and a radiologist interpretation. You perform x-rays and do not see an obvious foreign body. You are worried though, as the small intestine has two distinct populations. You see an area in the jejunum that is classically dilated (greater than two times the height of a lumbar vertebrae), and you are very worried about an obstruction. You discuss this concern with the owner and that you cannot confirm without further testing, surgery, or a second point in time. You go over the options with the owner, presenting them with multiple expensive estimates that include additional testing to further raise suspicion (barium study +/- abdominal ultrasound) vs. abdominal exploratory vs. hospitalization on intravenous fluids and repeat x-rays 8-12 hours later based on how the dog is doing clinically.

At this point in the process, many owners will feel anxious and confused. You have just thrown multiple expensive options at them without an exact diagnosis. All you have is suspicion, and as you can imagine from this scenario, it is not an easy conversation. Sometimes, all you can do is operate off of your gut instinct, physical exam, and "clear as mud" diagnostics. Just wait until you get an x-ray that you think is a slam dunk obstruction, and then it turns out to be a negative abdominal exploratory. In all of these cases, it comes down to the simple phrase of "to cut or not to cut." Your goal is to appropriately screen your cases to ensure your patients do not become a perforated surgical emergency. We are going to teach you how to guide these owners down the diagnostic pathway to ensure their pet is appropriately treated. So, where do you start?

Summary of your work-up plan

1. **Raise suspicion through a detailed history:** Ingestion? Exposure? Inability to hold anything down?
2. **Thorough physical exam:** Painful? Licking lips? Palpable object? Sick patient?
3. **Diagnostic plan:** 3 view abdominal +/- thoracic x-rays to raise suspicion.
4. **The great pretender:** Do not forget about systemic disease by performing blood work (CBC, chemistry, +/- cPLI) prior to surgery.
5. **To cut or not to cut:** Have a frank discussion on merit to further diagnostics vs. abdominal exploratory vs. hospitalization with repeat x-rays.

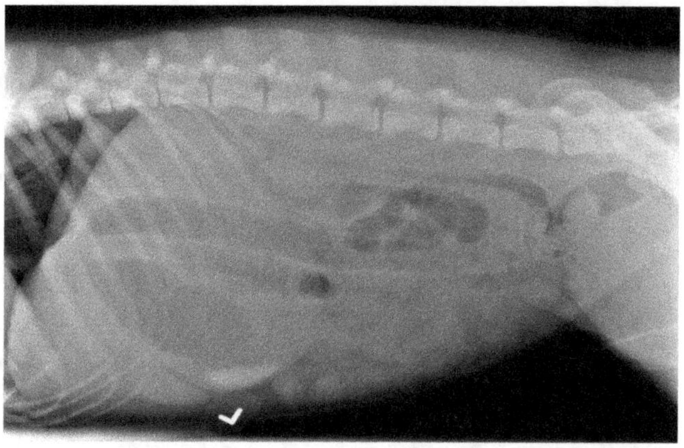

Patient presentation will be extremely variable. Your initial goal is to raise suspicion of a foreign body through your history and exam findings. **Common history findings that raise suspicion** are exposure, known ingestion, inability to hold down food +/- water, anorexia, lethargy, and profuse vomiting. Grill that owner about missing toys or chewed up household items like carpet, bedding, etc. Oftentimes, an owner's first reaction is no. We cannot tell you how many times we later hear "Oh, well he did chew up his leash or bedding last week" after further probing questions. Many owners do not think something that happened a few weeks ago, and sometimes MONTHS ago, could be the cause of today's issue.

Common physical exam findings include dehydration, ptyalism, abdominal pain (often they are very tense on palpation), palpable intra-abdominal foreign object, vomiting or regurgitating on abdominal palpation or in the room, licking lips, and lethargy. **One key point to remember is to always perform a thorough oral exam because many foreign objects can get lodged in the hard palate or around/under the tongue.**

Once you have suspicion of a foreign body, x-rays will be your starting point. The important thing to explain to an owner about an x-ray is that it is just one point in time, and it is not a 3D image. We like to tell an owner that x-rays raise suspicion in order to guide us toward our treatment options. Again, sometimes you get lucky and see an object on an x-ray. However, many times you do not, and instead see dilations or plication to raise suspicion.

Here is a very important tip with explaining x-rays to an owner that will benefit you in any case. You should be thorough when explaining x-ray findings to an owner because it will tell a lot about the pet's health. This pet may never have had an x-ray before. While they are there for one specific problem (vomiting), you should still tell them about everything you see, as it pertains to their health. Here are the steps we take when discussing an x-ray...

1. Start by explaining that you took a three view abdominal study (like a good veterinarian!). Use layman's terms such as this is a view of your pet laying on their side or back, instead of saying it is a lateral or V/D image, so the owner can understand what they are looking at.

2. Then, detail the findings that pertain to the primary concern. Point out the areas of concern as you talk about them because this will show the value to the owner.

3. Finally, explain other incidental findings like spondylosis or mineralization in the renal pelvis to be thorough but redirect them back to the main focus. This can be a quick blurb but is meant to help an owner in the future if they find other health issues develop, as you may not be their primary veterinarian.

This is an example of a spiel we use:

- *"Here, we have an x-ray of Sansa lying on her side. To put it in perspective, this is the area of her liver/stomach, here are her intestines, and in this area is her bladder and hips, so that you can have a rough idea of what you are looking at. I am worried about the dilation of her intestines in this area, as this can mean there is something blocking flow through her intestines, like a foreign object. While I know Sansa is here for vomiting, and I will touch on our plan shortly, I do want you to know about a few other findings, as these may be important later in life. I am seeing that she has some changes to her spine that fit with arthritis (spondylosis) as well as some mineralization in her kidneys that may make her prone to kidney disease in the future. While she is not here for this today, I want to make you aware of this for future visits. Any questions? Now, let's discuss our plan for Sansa today in order to improve her vomiting."*

Did you know there is a great pretender out there? Yes! Sometimes x-rays do not give you a clear cut answer, so you need to dig deeper with blood work as your next step. Some owners will not be open to performing both x-rays and blood work first due to cost, so be sure to explain its value when x-rays are in the "gray zone." Blood work will help you to complete the picture, and it will be needed anyways if surgery is indicated later. Our great pretender is **ileus**, which can be secondary to diseases such as pancreatitis, gastroenteritis, etc. You will see similar clinical signs, and it is a common cause of a negative exploratory. Atypical Addison's is another great pretender that has burned us before. Resting cortisol can be very useful here and help rule this out.

Therefore, ALWAYS be sure to run a CBC, chemistry, +/- cPLI after x-rays as your next diagnostic step after x-rays to be thorough.

Now, what? You will be presented with three common scenarios from your history, physical exam, and x-rays. We will discuss each here so that you can successfully guide your owners toward the best option.

You will be faced with these three scenarios most commonly

1. Obvious foreign body
2. Suspicion of partial or complete obstruction
3. Unclear

1. **Obvious foreign body:** These will be easy to diagnose, as you can show the owner the object of concern on your x-ray. You are now in a position of offering surgery or endoscopy as the best next step. Rarely, these will move with intravenous fluids. You run the risk of perforation or other complications with this option, but occasionally a sock or other soft item that is noted to be roughly in the distal jejunum may move along with intravenous fluids, if an owner is hesitant to go to surgery. These questionable sock-like foreign bodies can be started on intravenous fluids with the goal of close monitoring and repeat x-rays as a way to gauge progress. Always warn an owner of the possible complications with this "wait and see" approach. It can end up being more expensive if you end up needing to go to surgery later. When offering surgery, there are a few things to remember when communicating with your client.

    - **Provide an estimate range, like $2800-3500 for example, because these cases can become more complicated than a straightforward enterotomy.** This range will give you wiggle room if complications occur in surgery, more intensive surgery is required (such as an R&A), or if your patient needs to stay in the ICU longer to recover.

    - **Next, discuss complications. We keep it fairly simple stating that there are anesthetic complications that can occur such as low blood pressure, surgical complications like hemorrhage, immediate post-op complications like pain or GI upset, and complications at home like the incision opening up or getting infected.** Most owners will understand these complications, especially when asking for a code status. However, if needed, you can go into more detail on a case-by-case basis. Giving a few examples is enough, and you will be providing them with a surgery consent form they sign approving the procedure that will go into more detail as well.

- **Lastly, explain to the owner what they should expect while their pet is hospitalized.** This means a discussion on when the surgery will roughly take place, the treatments they will receive pre and post-op, and how you will be communicating with them. You can train your technician to do this too, but you want to make sure you leave the owner in a comfortable place where they know what to expect while their pet is in the hospital. It makes it less stressful for the owner, and it will save you multiple phone calls if the owner knows exactly what to expect from you. Our favorite phrase is "no news is good news" so that they are not extremely worried if surgery takes longer than expected or if you get caught up with other patients.

2. **Suspicion of partial or complete obstruction:** These cases will be difficult because it is not straightforward. Owners will waiver on how aggressive they want to be. You have a few options you can offer to your client in this situation.

    - **The first option is to perform additional diagnostics to get more information.** You can do a barium study, abdominal ultrasound, or even repeat x-rays 8-12 hours later (or sooner if the patient is not doing well). These additional tests may allow you to find the foreign body or help you feel better about the decision to offer in vs. outpatient care. This option is best for owners who are very against surgery or that want more information in order to choose the next best step.

    - **The second option is to hospitalize the patient on intravenous fluids with the goal of monitoring closely and performing repeat x-rays 8-12 hours later.** By keeping the patient in the hospital, you will be able to tell quickly if a patient is not responding well, which allows you to intervene sooner. If the patient is stable, this will allow you to get a second point in time with your x-rays to see if the dilation is the same, worsening, or improving. This option can make the estimate higher but will give you better confidence as to the next step.

    - **The third option is an abdominal exploratory.** Some owners feel very strongly that their pet ate something or just want to go forward with surgery, so it is always fair to offer this when there is a possibility of obstruction. You MUST warn them about the possibility of a negative exploratory. Prior to surgery, clearly explain that you have a plan A and plan B. Explaining these two plans allows you to move forward in the surgery based on what you find.

- ▽ **Plan A:** You find a foreign body and remove it. Have a discussion on the types of removal with gastrotomy, enterotomy, combination of each, and that sometimes unhealthy tissue needs to be removed too (R&A, for example). This is what causes variability in your estimate, as you never know what you need to do until you get into the abdomen.

- ▽ **Plan B:** Negative exploratory. Look, these are going to happen. When they do, prep the owner that biopsies will be an important next step. It is never a waste of time because it will help you understand why their pet is sick. You can sample the GI tract in different places along with any other grossly abnormal organs. Biopsies can be taken as either a wedge of tissue with an excisional technique, or we like using a punch biopsy.
    - ➔ **A note on negative exploratories.** We completely understand that you can end up beating yourself up when they happen, but we are here to remind you that it is going to happen at some point due to the imperfect nature of medicine. We make the best decisions we can with the information we have at that time. It is normal to feel disappointed with a negative explore but remember, it happens to even the best doctors and surgeons. No matter what, surgery will still help you to treat your patient appropriately, and you will also have your biopsies. The most important thing to do is to protect yourself to ensure the owner understands a negative exploratory is a possibility with these surgeries. Make sure the owner's are on the same page as you before going into surgery. We rarely have an upset owner regarding this because we communicate and make sure they understand this risk every time.

3. **Unclear diagnosis:** We should just go ahead and say it...these cases can really suck! In these situations, you do not have an exact diagnosis and are not confident about an obstruction. Offer further diagnostics like referral for an abdominal ultrasound and/or sending out a resting cortisol to look into other diseases that may cause similar clinical signs. These two tests have been invaluable and even helped prevent negative exploratories for us at times (which we discussed will happen!). If you have a very ill patient, you can also offer further diagnostics with hospitalization so you can assess their response to therapy. This

time in the hospital will allow you to adjust course based on their response, and repeat diagnostics.. If your patient is stable, you have a few options that we mention below, with the caveat that the owner needs to bring their pet back in if minimal improvement occurs or their pet declines.

Summary on what to do with your three most common FB scenarios

Obvious foreign body	Suspicion of partial or complete obstruction	Unclear diagnosis
▸ Great! You can visualize a foreign body in the GI tract. Now what? ▸ Abdominal exploratory or endoscopy will be your two best options. ▿ See above for all client communication points. ▸ Some "soft" foreign bodies (like socks) can be moved with intravenous fluids in those owners hesitant to perform surgery. Discuss risks and complications!	▸ Further diagnostics can be helpful in a stable patient (barium study, abdominal ultrasound, etc.) to get more information. ▸ Hospitalization and further diagnostics can be considered in an ill patient so that you can assess their response to therapy. ▸ When you offer abdominal exploratory, discuss Plan A and Plan B mentioned above. Some owners will want to just go to surgery.	▸ Further diagnostics can be helpful in a stable patient (barium study, abdominal ultrasound, resting cortisol etc.) to get more information. ▸ Hospitalization and further diagnostics can be considered in an ill patient so that you can also assess their response to therapy. ▸ Or consider outpatient care (mentioned below) in a stable patient with repeat x-rays 12-14 hours later to get a second point in time.

What if your owner is financially limited?

Unfortunately, this happens a lot in private practice. We separated this from the above options because this will be something you offer to anyone who is not immediately able to afford more than, let's say $500. Make sure you are up front with owners from the beginning that your exam and x-rays are just a starting point in order to determine what may be going on. Some owners will be up front and tell you they have financial limitations from the beginning. Others will not tell you until you have gone through your spiel above. **So, what do you do?**

- **Your first step is to provide your client with any payment options your hospital offers.** Care Credit and Scratch Pay provide clients with the ability to pay a larger bill over time, and it is simple to apply online. They will receive an approval within five minutes. This is a great time to utilize your receptionist to go over these options, as we strongly believe a veterinarian should be separated from more in-depth financial conversations. By separating you from the bill, we find clients tend to be more open with what they can do, and it separates your services from the cost so owners have time to process everything. Never forget that you have many other things you could be doing, so having your staff help with these conversations will free you up to write medical records, see other patients, etc.

- **Next, you can offer less aggressive treatment options if they are unable to apply for payment options, get declined, or if they do not have the financial means.** A caveat here...You MUST warn the owner that their pet may decline and become worse off (due to things like perforation). Mention to the owner that these options can mean a more expensive bill later, but sometimes these owners just really need time to figure out what to do, or they need time to work through finances. Their dog needs to be seen right away if they are not responding to these treatment plans at home.

    - **Option one** is fasting for 12 hours, subcutaneous fluids (¼-⅓ shock dose), and repeat x-rays 10-14 hours later as a comparison to x-rays in the "gray zone." This will help you feel more confident to confirm or deny an obstruction based on how your patient responded to treatment and by comparing your two x-ray studies.

    - **Option two** is fasting for 12 hours, subcutaneous fluids (¼-⅓ shock dose), and then the owner starts a bland diet the next day to see if their pet is able to hold down food. We will tell them to feed small amounts frequently while monitoring them closely the next 24-48 hours.

- **Unfortunately, if a patient continues to decompensate or follow-up exams indicate a surgical emergency, it is fair to offer euthanasia or owner surrender.** These options are extremely difficult, but if you know this patient will not get better, it is the most humane option for your patient. Surrender only works if you have a staff member or rescue willing to take over the medical care of the patient.

Tips from a boarded surgeon

Dr. Cleo Rogatko

- When setting up the table, I will save clean instruments in the back for closure.
- The stomach is often large and fluid or gas distended, so I'll usually have the tech pass an orogastric tube first to decompress it. Your initial gastric decompression can already get the pressure relieved on the intestines to get them healthier. Then, I'll generally leave an NG tube in place afterwards too. Aspirating contents post-op while recovering in hospital can help your patient feel much better and recover sooner. Like with a GDV, palpating NG tube for placement confirmation saves from the need to obtain post placement radiographs.
- If there is any free fluid in the abdomen, I will get a syringe and aspirate it. Half I will save in a culturette for culture and the other half I'll save for cytology. If it's a small amount and there is no intestinal perforation, look at it in-house and then if there is intracellular bacteria, commit to culture submission.
- I cut a hole in a blue drape if I'm going to do an enterotomy and I'll put the section of bowel through the hole to have a waterproof barrier to prevent contamination.
- Strelchik JAVMA 2019 found no difference in dehiscence rates between a simple continuous or simple interrupted closure for enterotomy, but usually I only do continuous if I have an assistant to run the suture and maintain significant tension on it between bites.
- Always count gauze.
- Always either take a picture of the foreign body removed or save it for the owner.
- Remember that you can break down the duodenocolic ligament with either cautery or metzenbaums to get more exposure of the distal duodenum at the flexure if needed.

NOTES:

NOTES:

Heart Murmurs in Small Breed Dogs

Reviewed by Dr. Jessica Romine, DVM, DACVIM

The majority of heart murmurs auscultated in small breed dogs are due to valvular disease (most commonly mitral valve disease). Though it is always important to involve a cardiologist if possible, many of these patients can be managed by general practitioners if the owner is unable to afford referral. Important things you can recommend for your small breed dog patients to keep tabs on their heart murmurs are routine exams, annual x-rays, and at home monitoring of resting respiratory rate. We are going to discuss our general recommendations, the "spiel" we give to owners, diagnostic tips, when to recommend referral, how to use medications, anesthetic tips, and more! This chapter will come in handy because the majority of your small breed senior patients will have some form of heart disease.

Diagnosing heart murmurs in patients

Hopefully you have had some practice listening to what heart murmurs actually sound like in clinics. It took us a lot of practice before we got comfortable hearing low grade heart murmurs, so do not fret if you are unsure if you hear one at times. Keep practicing and use the below tips to get better with time. If you ever have any doubt, just ask a colleague to listen or have a patient come back at another time for you to listen to it one more time. To this day, if we are not sure if we are hearing a murmur, we both *still* grab a colleague for a second quick listen. There is no shame in this! Remember, mitral valve murmurs are typically auscultated on the left side of the chest.

Some tips on auscultating heart murmurs

- For best results, have the animal standing and proceed in a systematic manner when listening to hearts. We often start at the left apex.
- Auscultate all valves every time and in the same order.
- Go to a quiet room with the patient if needed. This can make it easier to listen and helps them to keep still. *It can be very difficult to appreciate a subtle murmur in a busy treatment area!*
- Have your assistant gently hold the mouth closed if your patient is panting so that you can hear better.
- Do not forget to palpate femoral pulses while listening to the heart to assess for arrhythmias.
- **Tip from Dr. Jess for puppies or wiggly small dogs:** Try picking the dog up and carrying it around the hospital while walking swiftly. Auscultate at the same time *(you multi-tasking pro, you!)*, and the dog usually will stop wiggling around and vocalizing with this distraction. *Panting and whining can make our job hard, that's for sure!*

Talking to owners about a new heart murmur

This is one of those spiels you will wish you had recorded on video and could just play for an owner. We often find that many owners miss the concept the first time this is explained, so you may find yourself repeating it multiple times during other visits. It is important to note here as well that age of onset matters too. If you hear a murmur during a puppy or kitten visit and then it is still there by 6 months, it should be evaluated by a cardiologist if possible (or sooner if it is very loud). "Puppy/kitten" murmurs usually go away by 6 months. Below is our typical spiel to an owner. Yes, it is a mouthful!

Client communication summary for initial heart murmur diagnosis

- Your pet has a heart murmur. This indicates heart disease in dogs.
- Heart disease worsens with age.
- It is important we come up with a plan moving forward to monitor the heart murmur.
- Monitoring is done via thoracic x-rays, periodic echocardiograms, and resting respiratory rate.
- There are two main reasons for monitoring: timing of when to start medications and congestive heart failure.
- Medication will be warranted at some point to manage symptoms and improve heart function.
- Congestive heart failure will not develop in every patient. However, If it does develop, it can lead to death.

Here is how our conversation with a client goes

1. **Your pet has a new heart murmur:**

    a. *"Today, I can hear a heart murmur, which was not heard last visit. Have you ever had a pet with a heart murmur before?"*

        i. This can be helpful to know because an owner may already have some background information.

    a. *"In dogs, a heart murmur means there is underlying heart disease. And in a dog Fluffy's size, it is usually the valves of the heart that are diseased, meaning the valves are not opening or closing like they should."*

2. **The heart murmur can worsen with age:**

    a. *"As Fluffy ages, his heart disease will get worse and that means that Fluffy may have issues in the future with his heart function, even if he 'looks normal' on the outside.*

3. **Set up a monitoring plan and why we monitor it:**

a. *"We should consider setting up a plan to monitor his heart moving forward. There are two reasons we monitor heart disease. The first is to alert us as to when to start medication that can help him as there are key points in the progression of heart disease when we do this. The second is to be on the lookout for something called congestive heart failure which dogs with heart disease are prone to develop as the disease progresses. Congestive heart failure is a dangerous and life threatening condition where fluid builds up in their lungs and is something we need to keep close watch for as he ages.*

4. **Dose of perspective:**

    a. *"The good news is that many dogs can live for a long time before going on medications (months to years). Once on medications, prognosis can still be good, but I want you to understand that heart disease progresses at different rates. And though medications help the heart, it can still progress, which is why monitoring is so important."*

5. **The monitoring plan:** Let's talk about how we monitor heart disease.

    a. *"There are two ways we monitor this disease. The first way we monitor Fluffy is by getting some imaging or pictures of the heart done periodically. The best way to do this is through a cardiologist who can evaluate Fluffy's heart with an echocardiogram, which is an ultrasound of his heart. The next best option is starting with some baseline x-rays here with me to evaluate the heart size/shape, vessels, and lungs. We can always consider a cardiologist in the future if you do not wish to go initially. These two tests are helpful in allowing us to get a baseline on his heart function and if we do them periodically, we will find the right time to start Fluffy on medications that can help to prolong his life."*

        i. Offer every client all necessary diagnostics and the option of a cardiology consult the first time you hear a heart murmur. For those with financial concerns that decline referral or x-rays, focus on resting respiratory rate, monitoring of clinical signs, and semi-annual exams. Encourage them to save up for imaging. You need to continue to share with the owner the importance of why these tests are helpful each time you see them, especially if heart murmurs are getting louder.

b. *"The second tool we use is having you monitor his breathing rate at home. I am going to teach you how to monitor his breathing at home when he is sleeping, which is called the resting respiratory rate. This is VERY important because if he is breathing faster than normal, this can indicate fluid building up in his lungs. By monitoring his resting respiratory rate daily, you can pick up on problems before they become life threatening. If this does occur, medications will be needed to manage his heart disease."*

6. **Discuss resting respiratory rate:** Go over this with your owner so that they know how to monitor and track it. There are some great apps out there that clients can get on their phone to calculate it for them. The apps also store the data, so they can assess trends over time. Oftentimes, there is an option to email results to you too. Our favorite app is called Cardalis.

7. **Conclude and reiterate main points:**

   a. *"I know this is a lot to take in, but the most important takeaways from today are:*
      i. *Your pet now has heart disease. You don't need to modify his lifestyle at all just because he has a heart murmur. Exercise restriction isn't needed because he is not in heart failure, but now is the time to establish his "baseline" exercise tolerance and breathing rate so that you can pick up changes, and we don't want him to become sedentary and gain weight, which will only make the heart and lungs work harder.*
      ii. *We need to monitor it moving forward.*
      iii. *The way we do this is by counting a resting respiratory rate daily at home and performing chest x-rays with me annually +/- cardiology consult if able to financially (best to do annually as well)."*

8. **Lastly, always send handouts to go home.** Here are some of our favorites:

- Handout on heart disease (You can print one from Veterinary Partner).
- Resting respiratory rate sheet or discuss an app they can download (such as Cardalis).
- Information on referral to cardiology if the owner is open to going (prep them with cost).

Diagnostics for MVD

Here are a few key points to remember regarding two of the most common diagnostic tools you have in general practice for mitral valve disease. Remember, routine physical exams and monitoring resting respiratory rates are still going to be very useful when monitoring mitral valve disease long term.

We have a quick pro tip for you on performing diagnostics at this initial visit. **In general practice, it is easiest to set up the x-rays for another appointment time later that week**, as this discussion can take up a lot of your time. The other option is that they drop-off their pet for the diagnostics so that you can fit them in when able. By waiting for another day, it gives the owner some time to process what you have told them and allows you to answer any lingering questions when you call with the results later.

1. **Chest x-rays in regards to heart disease:** According to VIN and other sources, chest x-rays are:

    a. Moderately accurate in diagnosing left heart enlargement, especially when moderate to severe.

    b. Useful for diagnosing pulmonary edema. This is the hallmark of left sided congestive heart failure, though sometimes it is not apparent on x-rays right away.

    c. Can mean that you need to make your diagnosis based on history, clinical signs, physical exam, etc.

    d. Remember, when trying to distinguish primary lung vs. cardiac disease:

    e. Small breed dog + heart murmur + dyspnea + elevated proBNP ~90% accurate for diagnosing heart failure (Oyama 2009)

2. **Cardiac BNP basics:**

    a. Not good for diagnosing heart failure ALONE.

    b. Helpful in differentiating heart failure from lung disease in conjunction with physical exam findings and x-rays (see last point above about chest x-rays).

c. Can be helpful as a prognostic indicator. However, we often use chest x-rays to evaluate anesthetic candidates, as it is a better indicator of prognosis.

d. A plasma NT-proBNP concentration > 1,500 pmol/L, or a VHS > 12, or LVIDd:Ao > 3.0 indicates an increased risk for developing congestive heart failure within the subsequent 3 to 6 months (Oyama 2014).

e. BNP related to MST/median survival time (Moonarmart 2010)
   i. Dogs with an NT-proBNP concentration > 739 pmol/L (MST 318 days).
   ii. Dogs with an NT-proBNP concentration > 391 but ≤ 739 pmol/L (MST 786 days).

Treatment of MVD

The two most common times we are placing MVD dogs on medications are described below. Ideally, we would have 3 view chest x-rays at a minimum to support both of the findings mentioned below:

1. **Moderately enlarged left heart on x-ray or echocardiogram to start Pimobendan.**

   a. More specifically, we start it when the left atrium is 'at least moderately enlarged.'

   b. **Dr. Jess shares update:** A new review of the EPIC study, which originally showed that starting pimobendan delays the onset of heart failure, confirms its benefits. The review also suggests that starting pimobendan may be advantageous in dogs with a grade IV heart murmur, even if further diagnostics aren't possible.
      i. **Study to review:** Pegram C, Diaz-Ordaz K, Brodbelt DC, Chang Y-M, Boswood A, Wilshaw J, et al. Emulating the EPIC trial using VetCompass primary-care data: causal effects of pimobendan in UK dogs with grade IV/VI heart murmurs. PLoS One.2025;20(6):e0325695. Published June 18, 2025. doi:10.1371/journal.pone.0325695.
         1. The above study demonstrates that target trial emulation within veterinary research can replicate findings from RCTs. Clinically, the current findings suggest that preclinical grade IV murmur diagnosis may offer an appropriate intervention stage to begin pimobendan therapy in dogs with presumed DMVD.

2. **Congestive heart failure.**

   a. Most commonly we start our patients on furosemide, Pimobendan (if not already on it), and possibly spironolactone.

      i. ACE inhibitors are pretty out of favor with most cardiologists these days. They don't do very much for our patients and just add more cost and compliance issues with another medication to give a pet.

      ii. **New study alert from Dr. Jess:** A recent study looked at double therapy (pimobendan + furosemide) versus triple therapy (adding an ACE inhibitor) and quadruple therapy (adding spironolactone) in dogs with CHF. The study found no difference in survival. Before pimobendan was available, ACE inhibitors clearly improved survival compared to furosemide alone. But now, pimobendan is so effective that adding an ACE inhibitor doesn't seem to provide extra benefit. Due to this, most cardiologists are going back to double therapy with just pimobendan and furosemide because less is more! Spironolactone is still used if potassium drops, but otherwise, most dogs do well on just the two meds. A win for reducing pill burden in our CHF pups!

         1. Romito G, et al. Comparison of the effects of dual, triple, and quadruple medical therapy on cardiac death in a retrospective cohort of dogs with myxomatous mitral valve disease at American College of Veterinary Internal Medicine stage C: Is more necessarily better? J Am Vet Med Assoc. Published online 2025. doi:10.2460/javma.24.09.0588. Available at: https://avmajournals.avma.org/abstract/journals/javma/263/11/javma.24.09.0588.xml. Accessed January 25, 2026.

   b. Classic presentations for this include a dyspneic dog with a heart murmur or an elevated resting respiratory rate in a dyspneic dog with a heart murmur.

Furosemide trial? When and how?

Tip from Dr. Jess: If a dog is coughing intermittently, that is NOT an indication to do a furosemide trial. If it is congestive heart failure causing a cough, this is a wet, soft cough AND the respiratory rate should be increased with that much pulmonary edema going on. Our cardiologists see so many dogs put on furosemide for coughing when what they have is a heart murmur and bronchitis. X-rays can be very helpful here! Also, remember pulmonary crackles can be from chronic respiratory disease too, so it definitely doesn't mean automatic CHF.

Medications for MVD

1. Furosemide: This is THE drug you need for treating congestive heart failure (but not prior). This medication is a loop diuretic that treats fluid retention (edema) and swelling caused by congestive heart failure. It will be the medication you reach for to stabilize your congestive heart failure patient when they present unstable with dyspnea. Furosemide comes in oral tablets and an injectable form (5% or 50 mg/mL).

    a. Dose for acute heart failure: Furosemide: 2-4 mg/kg IV, IM, or SQ
        i. We usually start with 2 mg/kg IV as a bolus for those in respiratory distress. Titer upwards if needed depending on their response.
        ii. If hospitalizing, place in oxygen, monitor RR/RE, and repeat 1-4 mg/kg q6-8 hr or consider setting up a Lasix CRI if indicated. You are looking for an improvement in RR/RE over time.
            1. **Tip from Dr. Jess:** Our rule of thumb is when the respiratory rate comes down into the 30s, we start to reduce the rate and/or frequency of furosemide dosing.

    b. Dose for maintenance at home: 1-4 mg/kg PO q8-24 hr as needed. Again, we often start at 2 mg/kg PO BID if our patient is stable and renal/electrolyte values are normal.

    c. Furosemide tips:
        i. **Caution with kidneys:** Always warn the owner of the fact that the heart and kidney systems are usually "at war" with one another. While this drug may help the heart, it can hurt the kidneys too. Throughout the duration of

time their pet is on this drug, you will have to mitigate this the best you can through routine blood work screening 1-2 times yearly, based on what your owner can afford.

1. **Perspective from Dr. Jess:** Don't panic if the kidney values go up in acute CHF treatment. It doesn't automatically correlate with long-term outcome, but do remember to reduce down the furosemide as the acute exacerbation subsides.

ii. **Tailor dosage to the clinical signs and stability of your patient.** It is given to the patient more frequently when heart failure is present (q8-12 hr), and then once clinical signs have improved, you can consider decreasing to the lowest effective dosage. This should be done very carefully and slowly. Some dogs (especially repeat offenders), may not tolerate a dose decrease, while others will. Use diligent at home monitoring of resting respiratory rate by owners, consistent rechecks, and repeat x-rays as needed.

2. **Pimobendan:** Thanks to the EPIC study, pimobendan has been shown to prolong the life of mitral valve disease patients with moderate enlargement of the left atrium. This medication is a calcium sensitizer and selective inhibitor of phosphodiesterase 3 that has positive inotropic and vasodilatory effects.

   a. **Dose:** 0.25-0.3 mg/kg PO q12 hr.
      i. This dose is often increased to TID during later stages of heart disease.

   b. Start patients with moderate to severe enlargement of the left atrium on echo or chest x ray.

   c. If financial concerns prevent x-rays or diagnostics, and you have a patient with a severe heart murmur, use your best judgement on whether to start this medication. See above for more information about the EPIC study and further support about when to start medications.

3. **ACE inhibitors:** These medications produce vasodilation by inhibiting the formation of angiotensin II. This action helps to relax the blood vessels in order to lower blood pressure. Note: ACE inhibitors are beginning to lose favor in the management of CHF/MVD in dogs, as some cardiologists think it has little to no effect.

   a. **Doses:**

   i. **Enalapril:** 0.5 mg/kg PO q12 hr. It works best with BID dosing.
   ii. **Benazepril:** 0.25 mg/kg PO q24 hr. It works best with SID dosing.

b. It comes in an oral form.

c. Discontinue if you notice signs of uremia (clinical signs of renal insufficiency), as it could indicate low pressure in the glomerular system.

d. If able, it is ideal to check a kidney panel prior to starting this medication and 7-10 days later at your recheck to ensure it is well tolerated.

e. Studies of 2020 indicate there is no clinical need for its use prior to development of congestive heart failure. It has no effect on pre-clinical mitral valve disease.

When to recommend a cardiology referral

We always encourage referral when a heart murmur is first auscultated, but there are times when we will REALLY PUSH an owner to go to the cardiologist. These times are:

- There is a loud murmur present, and we have an anesthetic procedure we need to do. Yes, the grade of the murmur does not always correlate, but it is always better to be safe. If the owner still refuses and the pet needs the procedure, perform screening chest x-rays. Then, you can consider doing it as long as the owner understands the risk.

- We need to do anesthesia on a patient and have found concerning chest x-rays/cardiac BNP and/or resting respiratory rate. We want these dogs cleared before doing anesthesia.

- There is a chronic cough associated with their murmur. Think of pulmonary hypertension as a factor, and it can be difficult to manage without a cardiologist. The cough may also not be responding well to medications.

- A young adult dog with a heart murmur.

- A puppy with a continuous heart murmur or a murmur that does not resolve (or worsens) by 6-12 months of age, which increases concern for a congenital heart defect.

- New heart murmurs on pets fed at home diets that are NOT formulated by a boarded veterinary nutritionist or those on boutique, exotic protein, or grain free (BEG) diets.

- Cocker spaniels, which are a small breed that is also prone to DCM.

Anesthesia in dogs with heart murmurs

It can still be safe to perform anesthesia on patients with heart murmurs. You need to pick your cases wisely. If not overseen by a cardiologist, we recommend chest x-rays prior to assess for any signs of heart failure, heart enlargement, etc. If we do find an enlarged left atrium, we will likely still do the surgery but recommend starting the dog on Pimobendan first. We will also bring up the cardiologist one more time in case the owner is now open to an echo prior to anesthesia.

In general, for all dogs with heart murmurs, consider the following:

1. Always **recommend imaging** prior to any anesthetic event in a dog with a heart murmur. Document if they decline and ensure they know the risks involved.

2. **Pick your cases wisely** and use your best judgement! If you do not feel comfortable, you do not have to do the procedure. If you do, go over all risks and document everything!

3. Use a **benzodiazepine + opioid as their pre-medication**. Our favorite combination is midazolam + hydromorphone or butorphanol. We also use **maropitant** in all of our anesthesia patients to reduce nausea.

4. **Consider using Alfaxalone** instead of Propofol, since studies have shown Alfaxalone can be safer with heart disease. However, we have used both safely in patients with heart disease since Alfaxalone is not always readily available.

5. **Cut their fluid rate by half**, as maintenance fluid rates tend to be tolerated well.

As stated above, a dog with a loud heart murmur (grade 4-6) should be strongly recommended to have a cardiology consult. Your client may be more open to it since a procedure is now indicated for their pet. If the owner is not open to referral, you need to have a serious heart to heart with them about the risks involved with anesthesia.

Acute heart failure tips

Let's start with what an acute heart failure dog usually looks like: dyspneic with a historical heart murmur and crackles auscultated in the lung fields. When diagnosing dyspnea, assess the dog's chest and abdomen as they are breathing. **Is there an abdominal component? If yes, dyspnea!** We know it can be hard to accurately assess a panting dog's respiratory rate, so we find this trick is SUPER helpful.

Tips from Dr. Jess

STABILIZE first before diagnostics. If this patient is really dyspneic, you don't want to make a dog decompensate just to get an IV in or x-rays. Treat first with IM furosemide, oxygen, and butorphanol. Repeat based on response, and wait until they stabilize to get more information if you have to.

Your basic steps when triaging the small breed dog with dyspnea and a historical heart murmur:

- **Place on oxygen** right away. You can start with flow-by, so you can auscult your patient and get quick vitals. Focus on the important parts of your exam that are going to guide you in that moment. Then, put in an O2 cage if you have one, while you are talking with your owner to discuss what is going on. Mention to the owner the next few things you want to do to help their pet (with a rough cost) and that you will come back after the medications are administered to discuss next steps in more detail.
- **Administer furosemide 5%** (2-4 mg/kg SQ, IM, or IV). We will often give it IM to start, if we are unable to get quick venous access prior to doing anything.
- **Consider a dose of butorphanol** (0.2-0.3 mg/kg SQ, IM, or IV) to help your patient relax. Once butorphanol is kicking in, you should be able to get an IV catheter placed, if the owner is on board with therapy.

  - ▽ **Perspective from Dr. Jess:** Almost any dyspneic dog or cat will benefit from butorphanol. We give it right before they go into oxygen. It helps slow the panic component of dyspnea and is helpful whether it's respiratory or cardiac in origin.

- Have your **technician monitor the patient's vitals** while you are talking with the owner in order to assess when and if they are improving. Respiratory rate and effort are most important, as sometimes a second dose of furosemide can be administered 15-30 minutes later if it is unchanged.

- **Give a dose of Pimobendan orally** if your patient will tolerate it (once dyspnea has resolved from above treatments).

- **Pending stability of your patient, one diagnostic tool you can consider** to raise suspicion is POCUS. Oftentimes x-rays and bloodwork are unable to be performed for a few hours while your patient stabilizes, but you can fit in an efficient POCUS. You won't be able to position the dog perfectly, but see what views you can get to look for changes like an increased La:Ao ratio (large left atrium often a quick call you can make), b-lines, pleural or pericardial effusion, etc. We highly recommend getting additional ultrasound training to be able to do this in practice. It's a gamechanger!

- **Talk to the owners** about your concern for congestive heart failure, prognosis, and next steps. Oftentimes, you will not be able to do diagnostics right away because you have to stabilize your patient first. You cannot safely do x-rays until your patient's respiratory rate/effort and color has improved. Discuss your treatment plan to get their pet stabilized, cost, possible need for referral (if you do not work in a 24 hour facility), and the diagnostics needed (chest x-rays and blood work at a minimum).

LA:Ao Ratio

While the exact "normal" ratio varies, a value greater than 1.5-1.6 is generally considered dilated in dogs.

Initial client communication to owner with dyspneic small breed dog with presumed CHF

"Fluffy appears to be in respiratory distress, and she does not appear stable. I know she has a historical heart murmur, so I have some concern for congestive heart failure. This is where her heart is no longer able to keep up anymore, and her circulation is impaired. I have already placed her in an oxygen cage to help her feel better while we are talking. If you are ok with it, I would like to give her a dose of a diuretic, to help remove some fluid from her lungs, along with a medication that helps her heart work better. It will also help Fluffy to give her medication to help her relax, as this condition makes them feel very anxious. Is it ok if I check on her again, give her these three treatments, and then come back to talk to you about next steps?"

References:

- Oyama MA, Rush JE, Rozanski EA, et al. Assessment of serum N-terminal pro-B-type natriuretic peptide concentration for differentiation of congestive heart failure from primary respiratory tract disease as the cause of respiratory signs in dogs. J Am Vet Med Assoc 2009;235:1319–1325
- Moonarmart W Boswood A Luis Fuentes V, et al. N-terminal pro B-type natriuretic peptide and left ventricular diameter independently predict mortality in dogs with mitral valve disease. J Small Anim Pract 2010; 51: 84–96.

NOTES:

NOTES:

NOTES:

Hyperthyroidism in Cats

Reviewed by Dr. Jessica Romine, DVM, DACVIM

This is one of the EASIEST diseases to diagnose in cats. Whenever we are talking a cat owner into wellness bloodwork, we use hyperthyroidism as an example because it is the most common endocrine disease of cats. Getting an owner to "buy-in" to senior bloodwork works best by explaining the value they will get out of a test, as it relates to screening their cat for diseases. It is a very rewarding disease to diagnose because cats respond well to treatment, and they can often still live a long, healthy life.

So what's the deal with this disease?

Signalment: It is most common in senior cats >10 years old.

Common clinical signs: weight loss, muscle atrophy, diarrhea, vomiting, polyuria, polydipsia, polyphagia, hyperactive, weakness, irritability, vocalizing (especially at night), poor hair coat, tachycardia, arrhythmias (gallop most common), palpable thyroid nodule

Diagnosis:

- Test of choice is a total TT4.
- If in the gray zone with clinical signs (3.5-4, at upper end of reference range), you can run a free T4 as a confirmatory test.

Other abnormalities you may see:

- Elevated liver enzymes (ALT, AST, ALP)
- Azotemia (BUN, creatinine), though you may not see this until the cat is regulated on medications because hyperthyroidism can mask renal disease
- Hypertension
    - **From Dr. Jess:** HCM is often either caused by or exacerbated by hyperthyroidism (heart murmurs, even CHF) and sometimes can be reversed when effectively treated.

Treatment:

- Oral methimazole (2.5 mg and 5 mg tablet options) is the drug of choice. Dosing typically starts at 2.5 mg PO twice daily.
    - This drug can also be compounded into a liquid or transdermal* *(see below chart)* to be applied on the inner ear by a compounding pharmacy.
    - Side effects are rare, but we always warn owners of blood work abnormalities and facial pruritus
- Hill's Y/D diet
    - We tend to only use this diet when other treatments are NOT an option (ex: methimazole reaction) or the "borderline cats" that have a TT4 between 3-5, as we do not find it drops the value much.
    - You cannot use it in a multi cat household or in homes where a cat has access to ANY other foods by mouth (dog food or human food). If not strict, it does NOT work!
- Surgery (thyroidectomy)
    - Curative option
- Radioactive iodine therapy
    - Curative option
    - Considered the gold standard and preferable if owners will pursue
    - The biggest con is that in rare cases it can cause hypothyroidism, which would need to be treated with medication for life. Before referral**, look at requirements to make sure your patient is a good fit!

*Dr. Jess Treatment Notes:

Transdermal Methimazole: transdermal methimazole seems to eventually work as well as oral methimazole, but it takes longer to reach efficacy. So if you have a pretty symptomatic cat, start with oral if possible. It can take up to 6 weeks to reach steady state with transdermal vs. 2-3 weeks with oral.

Radioactive Iodine: With this treatment, they do have to be kept in a protected cat ward until they are not radioactive afterwards, so animals do need to be stable. You can underdose and have to repeat as well (generally about 5% of cases). I LOVE I 131 because it's a spectacularly effective option in most cases, and it's not horribly expensive, especially if you compare it to the cost of monitoring and medications for oral medications for life. It is definitely worth discussing with owners, even if they don't go right away. Start on methimazole and give pricing/ wait times for your area for 131 (probably about $1500-$2000), and encourage them to start saving towards it if they have any interest.

There are a few things you should be aware of with this disease. Thyroid disease can cause other diseases or be found concurrently with underlying hypertrophic cardiomyopathy, for example. You may also find kidney disease (especially once hyperthyroidism is managed because treatment can unmask it), heart disease, and hypertension. It is important to be thorough and rule all of these secondary diseases out once you know a cat has hyperthyroidism. Oftentimes, if you catch hyperthyroidism in the early stages, you can minimize injury to other organs. That right there will sell many owners on bloodwork every 6-12 months. These other diseases can mean a poorer prognosis.

So, you diagnose hyperthyroidism in a cat. Now, what should you tell the owner?

Client communication points:

- ake sure to **discuss ALL treatment options** with the owner when you first diagnose their cat. The cheapest option will always be medical management, but some owners may want a more permanent solution. As we know, medicating cats can be difficult, so we find owners can warm up to the idea of radioactive iodine over time if they struggle to medicate their cat.

- **If an owner chooses medical management**, do not forget to go over the side effects of methimazole. Honestly, you need to get in the habit of doing this for every drug you give a patient in order to prevent a client complaint.

  - **Common side effects to mention include** anorexia, lethargy, vomiting, diarrhea, facial pruritus, and bone marrow dysfunction/low white cells/anemia.
    - **Tip from Dr. Jess:** Cats that get GI upset on the oral methimazole can often tolerate transdermal instead. However, if they get facial itching or bone marrow issues on oral, they will also get this on transdermal, so you'll have to consider other options.

  - Do not forget to mention that with medical management, their cat will never be cured, only managed. The medication blocks the synthesis of thyroid hormone.

- If an owner is interested in surgery or radioactive iodine, contact your local facility to determine what you need to do prior to referral. Oftentimes, you still need to start medical management in order to get the cat stabilized. We know many referral facilities also want you to repeat a TT4 prior, as well as other tests like a urinalysis. They do not want concurrent infection, so talk with your local specialist to ensure the referral process is smooth.

- If an owner opts to change formulation, such as going from an oral tablet to transdermal, warn them that you will need to recheck TT4 again 3-4 weeks after the change. Sometimes, transdermal does not absorb as well, and cats may need a higher dosage. Transdermal can take up to 4 weeks to start working.

- Prepare an owner that sometimes another disease can be unmasked after stabilizing the cat's thyroid levels. We often see normal kidney values initially with uncontrolled hyperthyroidism, then once it is controlled, kidney disease is unmasked. This will be important because we do not always recheck kidney values, but if an owner wants to be thorough, you can do this the same time as the recheck TT4. Early intervention is always key to ensuring we are doing everything we can for their cat to keep them healthy as long as possible.

- If you have a borderline hyperthyroid cat that has a TT4 in the upper end of the reference range and normal fT4, make sure you can palpate a thyroid nodule (thyroid slip test). If so, recommend that they come back in 6 months to recheck sooner than their annual, as they are most likely still developing the disease. You have just not caught it yet.

Recheck plan: **Recheck TT4 in 2-4 weeks** to ensure medical management is appropriate. **Dose should be in the mid-normal range.**

- A good approach to take with an owner when discussing a recheck of any endocrine disease is that you do not want to cause the opposite disease. Over-supplementing can occur, and sometimes it can take a few dose adjustments to find the right amount for their cat.
    - From Dr. Jess: This is important because hypothyroidism causes worsening kidney disease, so you don't want to do this to a senior cat!

- If an owner is "gung-ho" and not financially limited, it is always ideal to repeat a CBC and chemistry with their TT4 to see if we have unmasked kidney disease, as well as to ensure prior liver enzyme elevations have improved. Rarely, hepatopathy can develop after starting methimazole. Blood pressure can also be important to do at this stage.

- Just remember, you will have a wide variety of clientele. Always give each client the "spiel", but you will need to offer a range of care based on what an owner can afford. If an owner can only do the bare minimum, focus on what is most important.

Hyperthyroid disease in cats summary

1. **Diagnosis:** elevated TT4 above reference range, palpable thyroid nodule, and clinical signs = hyperthyroidism.

2. **Screen for concurrent disease** such as kidney disease, hypertension, cardiac disease, etc., which may not be apparent until after treatment.

3. **Discuss treatment options** and pick the best plan for the patient and owner.

4. **Recheck in 2-4 weeks** with a TT4 along with a CBC, chemistry, and blood pressure if cost allows. Continue rechecks until appropriate dosage is found.

5. **Long term recheck plan** is semi-annual exams and blood work every 6-12 months (CBC, chemistry, T4,.UA) based on what an owner can afford.

NOTES:

NOTES:

Lick Granulomas in Dogs

Reviewed by Dr. Jeff Tinsley, DVM, DACVD

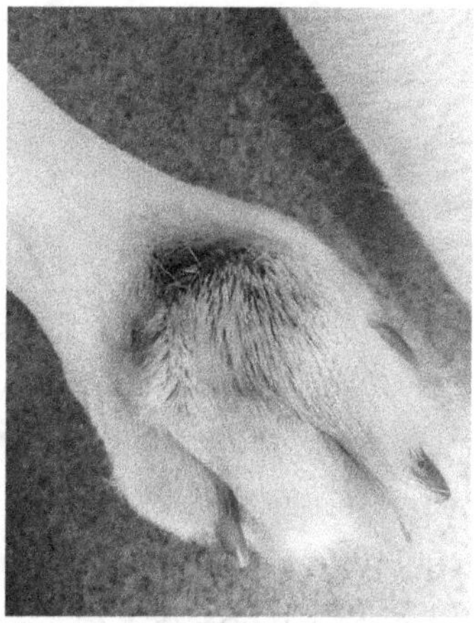

What is a lick granuloma? Lick granulomas are thickened, raised, sometimes nodular areas of skin that are always secondary to one or more underlying causes. The underlying trigger leads to constant lick response from the dog with subsequent inflammation and thickening of the skin. They routinely incur a secondary, deep bacterial infection.

Lick granulomas may not seem like a big deal....until you get a client complaint about the never ending sore on their dog's leg that you have failed to resolve. This is a disease where **communicating chronicity** and **expectations** is VITAL to a successful outcome and forming trust with your client. Here is how we do it.

First, how do you differentiate a lick granuloma from something else? Well, history will be very important here. These lesions form due to chronic licking where the pet fixates on a specific area. The most commonly affected areas are the front limbs between the elbow and toes.

Underlying causes to consider:

- Allergies
- Psychogenic/OCD behavior
- Boredom
- Cutaneous foreign body
- Licking due to pain/arthritis
- Infectious (demodex, ringworm, etc.)
- Neoplasia
- And more

Client communication points:

1. From the start, **communicate that these are frustrating and difficult to treat:** Set your owner up with this expectation. These do not resolve without time, proper management at home, and often can recur if the underlying cause is not managed appropriately throughout their lives.

2. **Underlying cause:** Try to determine your underlying cause because this will guide your treatment plan along with the strategies for prevention. Allergies are often the most common cause, but occasionally dogs can develop behavioral dermatoses (such as an "OCD" component) or constant licking due to pain.

Some tips from Dr. Jeff

- It is appropriate to rule out allergies first if the history fits (see our chapter on pruritus for some tips on how to manage underlying allergies). Most of these cases will begin with a history of licking prior to lesions occurring and the pruritus is typically multifocal.
- If the owner thinks the lesion (in this case a lick granuloma) was spontaneous, then allergies may be less likely. For example: the owner saw the nodular area first and the patient has never exhibited prior pruritus but is constantly licking at a single focal area. Ruling out differentials like Demodex, dermatophytosis, foreign body, etc. first are indicated.
- If the history involves a possible injury or the dog runs or hunts on lots of land, then consider ruling out a foreign body. Radiographs may be beneficial. A 2 week NSAID pain med trial to assess for soft-tissue injury or work-up for arthritic pain may be warranted.

3. **Long term antibiotics:** These patients often **need to be on antibiotics for a minimum of 6-8 weeks,** and sometimes 8-12 weeks in tough cases, as a deep secondary bacterial infection is nearly always present. Due to the length of course needed for treating deep infection, it is recommended to perform skin cytology and offer culture and sensitivity of these cases. For best culture results, a biopsy punch is collected (under sedation), macerated and submitted. If you're unsure of the underlying etiology, a biopsy punch sample can also be submitted for histopathology. To prioritize deep bacteria for the culture, many

dermatologists will sanitize the skin surface with alcohol and some remove the top layer of the epidermis with a 10-blade prior to culture/sensitivity submission.

- Dr. Jeff wanted to share that if a client declines is not ready for deep tissue culture, it is appropriate to begin with first line empirical antibiotics for 4 weeks, and then re-assess. If the lesion greatly responds, continue the antibiotics for another month and re-assess. If not improving at any recheck, then it's culture time!

4. **Even if the dog licks the paw for just a minute or two, the infection will persist, and it will never heal:** CONVEYING THE IMPORTANCE OF THIS TO THE OWNER cannot be overstated. Keeping the dog from licking the paw is absolutely necessary for improvement of this condition. We have healed these completely, and then the dog licks for a few days, which puts us back to square one. Just one minute of licking can set the dog back weeks. Options include use of an e-collar, dog clothing (if it will cover well), and/or www.dogleggs.com for protective wear that covers it.

5. **Use a combination of the below treatment options** in order to heal a lick granuloma. You can always start with an initial plan and add on over time based on response.

Initial diagnostics to guide your treatment plan:

1. Skin scrape
2. Skin cytology
3. +/- Skin culture and sensitivity

Lick granuloma treatment guide

- **Long term antibiotics:** (6-8 weeks minimum): cephalexin, cefpodoxime, or clindamycin work very well. Remember, often deep infection is present. A tissue culture and sensitivity is always preferred due to the expected length of treatment.

- **Long term anti-itch medication:** If you believe the case fits with allergic pruritus, it will likely require long-term maintenance with antipruritics. See the pruritus and allergy chapter for more details and full workup recommendations. During lick granuloma treatments: minor lesions may benefit from Apoquel, more severe lesions often require steroids like prednisone to resolve. These medications both have some anti-inflammatory properties which are important as most lick granulomas have inflammation within the skin. Cytopoint exclusively helps with pruritus and not inflammation, therefore is best reserved for antipruritic use once the lick granuloma has resolved.

- **E-collar or other protective covering:** You will find that clients always want to try socks or at home bandages. We find these are often ineffective, as they just lick on top of the sock, and it does not do anything. If a client wants to do this, warn them that you have seen some dogs eat bandages, so they understand the risk. Try to find the best e-collar option–there are many innovative ones out there now!

- **Topical treatment:** These can also be very helpful. Initially, a topical steroid like Synotic, Animax or other ear-based ointment containing a steroid can be beneficial. Be aware that use of topical steroids on the skin for more than 14 days is generally discouraged to prevent unwanted thinning of the skin. A chlorhexidine based mousse like Douxo S3 Pyo Mousse can be used as well. However, these should be used in conjunction with systemic anti-inflammatories and antimicrobials since they may not penetrate deeply into the tissue.

- **Flea/Tick prevention:** An isoxazoline product (Bravecto, Simparica, Nexgard, or Credelio) is recommended to cover for Demodex. If starting an elimination diet trial, you can consider the topical formulation of Bravecto. The chewable version is OK exclusively at the beginning of a diet trial.

- **Phovia therapy:** This is a newer technology that Dr. Jeff wanted to share more information on. Phovia is photobiomodulation with fluorescent light and has been shown to resolve pyotraumatic dermatitis. It has antimicrobial and anti-inflammatory properties. It is non-invasive. It may require several sessions for efficacy. Anecdotally, some clinicians use this for 3-4 weeks to assess efficacy.

- **Laser therapy:** If you have a cold laser at your hospital, daily laser therapy has been shown to improve healing time with many acute or chronic wounds. There are many protocols, but a common one is daily for 7 days then every 2-3 days, until healed, or nearly healed. The length of time is determined by the machine when you type in the location, size, etc.

- ▽ Dr. Jeff hasn't seen much success with lasers specifically for lick granulomas, but Ashley and Monica have used laser therapy with success. It is worth a try if you have a willing owner and one in your hospital.

- **Rechecks every 3-4 weeks:** This will depend on your estimation of client compliance. We find 4 and 8 weeks are good time frames, as it allows you to adjust therapy based on response. These take time to heal, so you need to see it at different stages to note progress and to keep the owner motivated with treatment.

- **Elimination diet trial (8 weeks minimum on strict Rx diet):** If the case fits with allergy and exhibits nonseasonal pruritus, this is an important thing to mention on Day 1, even if the owner opts to pursue it on a recheck visit. If your client is not open to the idea yet, we make sure they understand that this is our next step if pruritus leads to lick granulomas recurrence. If you do an elimination diet trial, here are some parasite preventative combinations you can try that will not interfere.

  - ▽ Bravecto + Revolution: Although Bravecto is hydrolyzed pork, it is preferred to avoid in the middle of a diet trial, but OK to give at the start of a diet trial. . There is also a topical Bravecto. It should cover Demodex too! Revolution is a topical.

  - ▽ Topical flea/tick option (Vectra-3D, Activyl, Bravecto topical, etc.) + Proheart injectable

- **Reduce boredom:** Have clients try to increase activity to reduce boredom, which can promote licking. This can look like 2-4 walks per day. Short, frequent walks may be best if they are not a highly active breed. An owner can also offer daily Kongs with canned food or peanut butter to lick instead of their arm, 15 minute training sessions daily, puzzle toys, etc.

- **Stress reduction tips from Dr. Jeff:** For suspect high anxiety leading to skin lesions/lick granulomas, identify and reduce sources of stress in the home. Some cases may benefit from 2-3 month trials of medication-based behavioral modifiers like SSRIs. Some cases also benefit from consults with a board-certified veterinary behavior specialist. This is especially important if they are progressive with recurrent, non-resolving problems and allergy has been ruled out.

Extra tips for lick granulomas

- **Take pictures,** attach to your patient file and measure the lesions. This will help you remember exactly how it looked so that you can objectively compare diameter size at each recheck. This can also be helpful if an owner does not feel it is healing, as you can show them the picture and measurement progress.

- **Send home with a handout.** We ALWAYS give owners a handout eliciting the points we make so that the plan is clearly stated for best compliance. It is easy for them to miss a point or forget one, as there are several things that they have to understand. You can also state next steps at the end of the handout if it does not improve such as an elimination diet trial, relaxant medications like trazodone, pain medications like gabapentin, or a dermatology consult for environmental allergy testing.

- **Culture (w/ sensitivity) when possible.** Let the client know that if an infection persists, a tissue culture is the next step (if not pursued on initial exam). Prep them with the price. The most ideal way to collect your culture sample is to sedate your patient and get a biopsy punch sample of tissue to send off because the infection is typically deep.

- **Give them the option of a dermatology referral** if the lick granuloma is not responding as you expect. We always mention that if they ever want to go to a dermatologist to just let our office know. It is important to show that you are always open to collaboration and a second opinion. It builds trust.

References:

- Muller, George H., et al. Muller & Kirk's Small Animal Dermatology. 7th ed., Elsevier, 2013.
- Luciani L, Marchegiani A. "Photobiomodulation with fluorescent light energy as a sole treatment of pyotraumatic dermatitis (hot spot): a case series" J Am Vet Med Assoc. 2025, doi.org/10.2460/javma.24.12.0820

NOTES:

NOTES:

Osteoarthritis in Dogs

Reviewed by Dr. Gabriella Varcoe, DVM, DACVSMR, CCRP

Osteoarthritis can (and does) occur at any age. We have both seen two year old dogs present with chronic lameness due to arthritis that developed at an early age. We have both euthanized dogs due to mobility issues. We have both seen pets in chronic pain where the owner is resistant to medical management. These cases can be difficult for both the owner and you as the veterinarian because expectations can vary. Some owners will be on board with trying anything, while others will be resistant to any therapy options you offer.

So, what is the best approach for your young and old patients? How will you communicate the importance of arthritis management in your middle aged to senior pets? We are here to share our approach with you, as we dish our random tips, drug protocols, alternative therapies, favorite management strategies, and more!

Classic phrases you will hear from owners about pets with arthritis

- "My dog is not able to jump up on his favorite couch as gracefully as he once could."
- "My dog seems a little stiff in the morning but warms up after a while."
- "My dog still plays but not as much as she used too."
- "My dog sleeps all the time and used to be active."
- "My dog struggles to get up from laying down."
- "My dog is sitting weird."

Client communication basics

Here are some points you want to ensure you get across to owners.

- Arthritis is a degenerative joint process that will continue to occur over their life.
- Arthritis leads to inflammation in the joints, which is the main source of acute or chronic pain. It helps to relate these symptoms to human medicine, as many owners have arthritis or chronic pain as well.
- Lameness will be a common presenting complaint that you will see in general practice. Outside of lameness, dogs cannot easily tell us about their chronic pain, so it is important to analyze any behavior changes closely. We also stress to owners to bring them in for clinical signs that seem off from their normal routine.
- Recommend to the owner that they consider starting therapy sooner rather than later. The goal is to manage arthritis early in order to slow down the process of cartilage degeneration. Your treatment is aimed at slowing and decreasing the inflammatory cascade and stress on the joints as much as possible. By being proactive, the owner can slow down the progression of arthritis.
    - **Dr. Gabby Insight:** Many times by the time some of these interventions are instituted we are already too late. Early-onset OA is often secondary to hip/elbow dysplasia, trauma, or OCD (osteochondritis dissecans).
- Recommend x-rays for lamenesses that are recurrent or not improving with exercise restriction and NSAID therapy.

Random tips

- Tip 1: When taking an x-ray of a limb, always take the opposite limb for comparison, **take more than one view of each joint** (including orthogonal views).
- Tip 2: Do not forget to check for neck and back pain, as forelimb lameness can often be due to neck pain.
- Tip 3: Do not fight with your patient. Sedation is your best friend, especially if surgery may be indicated so that you can get the appropriate views.

Dr. Gabby Tip

It's important to use validated pain scales, like the CBPI, with your clients to establish a baseline and track progress during rechecks. There are several good options available that can be sent home with them.

For every pet with suspected arthritis or mobility issues, recommend:

1. **Keep your pet lean.** We like a BCS of 4/9. Explain to owners that this is the single most important thing they can do for their pet. Help their goal be attainable by giving them a calorie count and diet suggestion for weight loss. We recommend monthly weigh-ins with nurse appointments to help them remain accountable and keep track of their goals. This approach allows you to adjust the plan if it is not working.

    a. Some great diet options are Purina Pro Plan OM Metabolic Response + Joint Mobility and Hill's Metabolic Mobility. We love these two options because they function as both weight loss diets AND are formulated with joint supplements. You can find strictly joint diets out there if your patient is already at ideal BCS. If their dog will not eat those diets, you can try traditional weight loss foods like Purina Pro Plan Weight Management, Purina OM, Hill's Metabolic, or Royal Canin Satiety.

        i. Dr. Ashley's dog has been on Purina OM/JM for years now and has maintained great mobility and his weight, despite routinely vacuuming up toddler morsels. He is horrible at taking medications so having the supplement within the food is a great option for tough to pill pets or forgetful pet parents.

Monitoring weight, muscle, and joint health in dogs *from Dr. Gabby*

- **Body condition score (BCS)**
  - It is recommended to use a **validated body condition scoring (BCS)** system to assess overall body fat. WSAVA provides excellent charts for client education: WSAVA BCS Charts.
  - Visual aids are very helpful for owners. During appointments, showing the chart and reviewing the dog's current score with the owner improves understanding and engagement.

- **Muscle condition score (MCS)**
  - In addition to BCS, it is important to assess **muscle condition score (MCS)**. Muscle loss (sarcopenia) often accompanies osteoarthritis (OA) and can impact mobility and quality of life.
  - WSAVA also provides MCS charts for client education: WSAVA MCS Charts.
  - Tracking MCS allows you to monitor lean muscle over time, especially during weight management or in older dogs.

- **Objective measurements**
  - For overweight or obese patients, **thoracic and abdominal circumference** measurements using a tape measure can provide objective data beyond body weight.
  - Recording these measurements at the initial consult and during rechecks can be motivating for owners, as improvement may be seen even if weight changes slowly.

- **Feeding and portioning**
  - Accurate portion control is critical. Using a **food scale** provides the most precise measurement of intake.
  - If using measuring cups, providing a physical cup for reference can help owners visualize the correct portion size. Many owners are surprised at how much a cup actually contains.
  - Some patients may require adjustments to their feeding plan if weight loss is insufficient with the current diet.

- **Nutritional considerations**
  - Ensure dogs receive **adequate protein**, particularly older dogs, to preserve lean muscle mass during weight loss.
  - Avoid overly rapid weight loss, as this can reduce muscle mass and negatively impact overall health.

- **Summary**
  - Combine **BCS, MCS, and circumference measurements** to track progress objectively.
  - Use **visual tools and client education** to support owner engagement and compliance.
  - Adjust **diet and feeding strategies** thoughtfully to promote safe, gradual weight loss while maintaining lean muscle and supporting joint health.

2. **Transition to low impact exercise as a way of life.** Exercise must be consistent and daily. Arthritic joints need movement but not stress. Explain to the owner with the dog that likes to chase balls to instead go on long walks with his ball or do short tosses in the yard. If their dog likes to swim, this is another great option for their dog. Decrease use of stairs and have them limit pets from jumping on and off furniture.

    a. If the owner is able to take it a step further, rehabilitation therapy is a great modality to assist orthopedic conditions in dogs. They can go to a facility that specializes in this, ensuring the dog gets a mix of underwater treadmill exercise, balance therapy, obstacle courses, etc. You can also incorporate exercise plans for your patients where owners take their dogs up and down hills, do short but frequent walks to build over time, and more. The goal here is to improve muscle mass.

3. **Supplements and medications:**

    a. **Omega 3 fatty acids:**

        i. **Suggested Dose:** the optimal dose has not been determined but we use 40 mg/kg/day eicosapentaenoic acid (EPA) and 25 mg/kg/day docosahexaenoic acid (DHA). There are many doses you can use, but this is just one we use. Most dog foods will not have this much unless it is a prescription joint diet.

1. **Note:** When you add this supplement in, be mindful of the amount of calories it adds with some products. It is also important to warn owners that its sudden addition can cause diarrhea in some dogs. We will often tell owners to start with every other day administration for a few weeks, then increase to daily when they note normal stools.

ii. It should be deep sea fish based, so we recommend it come from a company with good quality control. It is also helpful if it contains vitamin E as an anti-oxidant too.

iii. Avoid cod liver and plant based fish oils.

1. Why? Avoid cod liver oil because it has high concentrations of vitamin A and D, which can result in toxicity. Plant based are inefficient in dogs due to minimal elongation of a-linolenic acid (ALA) to EPA and DHA and ALA is minimally converted in dogs and cats.

iv. **Over-the-counter products we recommend:** Veterinary Recommended Solutions (VRS), Nordic Naturals, and Freeform Omega Fatty Acid

1. **Dr. Gabby Insight:** Small fish are better, salmon tends to accumulate heavy metals and other toxins due to longer lifespan. Most of the studies done on fish oils have been using diets enriched with therapy levels, however, adding in fish oil is something I recommend for my OA patients so they do not need to use a therapeutic diet if they don't want to (diets tends to be better tolerated, some dogs do not tolerate full dose fish oils when added (stomach upset).

b. **UC II (Flexadin Advanced):**

i. There is more research behind the efficacy of this supplement than glucosamine. It is in Flexadin Advanced (not Flexadin plus). It can be used with omega 3's.

ii. It is not recommended to use with glucosamine, as it decreases efficacy (*Gupta paper).

c. **Glucosamine:**

i. There is little evidence that glucosamine works. However, we do have some patients that seem to respond to it based on the owner's interpretation. Consider placebo effect, which can be 40% in owners (and higher in vets!)

- Conzemius MG, Evans RB. Caregiver placebo effect for dogs with lameness from osteoarthritis. J Am Vet Med Assoc. 2012 Nov 15;241(10):1314-9. doi: 10.2460/javma.241.10.1314. PMID: 23113523.

ii. There is more evidence supporting avocado/soybean unsaponifiables (ASU), so if you do recommend glucosamine, Dasuquin is a reasonable option because it has extra ingredients in it.

iii. If the owner is insistent on an over-the-counter version, you can recommend Cosequin, which is just plain glucosamine and chondroitin. Most glucosamine products take about 4-6 weeks to work, due to needing a loading dose, where an owner notices a difference.

d. **Adequan (polysulfated glycosaminoglycan):**

i. This injection is one of our favorites! It is the only FDA approved disease-modifying osteoarthritis drug. It inhibits cartilage loss in the dog's joints, which may help to restore joint lubrication, relieve inflammation, and renew the building blocks of healthy cartilage. (information taken from adequancanine.com).

ii. It works best to start it at the first signs of arthritis and then to stick with it in management long term.

iii. You can teach some owners how to give it at home to decrease stress on your patient. Off label, most vets will teach owners to give it subcutaneously, instead of intramuscularly.

e. **CBD (cannabidiol):**

i. At the time of our publishing (early 2026), there is promising data that CBD's can be helpful in management of arthritis. It is still not accepted by the AVMA that we recommend it for our patients, so it is a "fine line" right now where we can mention its use. Let owners know that it is important to find a good source if purchasing for their pet and that they can use it "off label at their own risk." Many companies are doing research on it, as we speak, which is great.

ii. Many of the current CBD products for pets have poor quality control, uncertain ingredients, and are poorly regulated as a whole.

iii. Encourage the choice of products with independent laboratory testing and certificate of analysis on their products (Example: Ellevets and Chroniquin, which is made by a Nutramax subsidiary). There are also local compounding pharmacies making their own treats for owners.

Dr. Gabby Tip on CBD

Note that studies have shown elevations in Alk Phos. Get baseline blood work prior. Also look for companies that do 3rd party testing. Hemp can accumulate a lot of pesticides etc from the soil so they should have a certificate of analysis. You also want a well rounded product, not just CBD, and caution with THC. Companies should test for multiple forms of THC when doing the certificate of analysis, not just the delta-9. Look for products with a certificate of analysis that verifies low THC levels (under 0.3%) and confirm the actual CBD content.

In general, you need to consider multiple things when choosing (and avoid human products):

- how was it grown, is it organic?
- 3rd party tested?
- How was the product extracted?
- Is the company reputable, have they done clinical trials in the species intended for its use?

Wakshlag JJ, Cital S, Eaton SJ, Prussin R, Hudalla C. Cannabinoid, Terpene, and Heavy Metal Analysis of 29 Over-the-Counter Commercial Veterinary Hemp Supplements. Vet Med (Auckl). 2020 Apr 15;11:45-55. doi: 10.2147/VMRR.S248712. PMID: 32346530; PMCID: PMC7169471.

Spindle TR, Sholler DJ, Cone EJ, Murphy TP, ElSohly M, Winecker RE, Flegel RR, Bonn-Miller MO, Vandrey R. Cannabinoid Content and Label Accuracy of Hemp-Derived Topical Products Available Online and at National Retail Stores. JAMA Netw Open. 2022 Jul 1;5(7):e2223019. doi: 10.1001/jamanetworkopen.2022.23019. PMID: 35857320; PMCID: PMC9301515.

Front. Vet. Sci., 29 February 2024

Sec. Veterinary Pharmacology and Toxicology

Volume 11 - 2024 | https://doi.org/10.3389/fvets.2024.1349590

f. **Gabapentin:**
   i. This is a drug in the anticonvulsant class that helps treat neuropathic pain. It works by decreasing the release of excitatory neurotransmitters.
   ii. Most of the specialists in our area prefer for owners to try this prior to daily NSAIDs due to the potential long term effects with chronic NSAID therapy. However, it is a great complement to an NSAID because it works through a different pathway.
   iii. This drug is helpful for many dogs, however, some owners do not like it. The main complaints are that it causes their dog to be sleepy or that owners do not think it is working well. If it causes drowsiness, try to adjust the dose lower or try an NSAID instead.

g. **NSAIDs:**
   i. This will be one of your most effective drugs for decreasing joint inflammation. Though there are some chronic side effects with its usage, it does tend to work very well.
   ii. Examples of products in this category that we like are Rimadyl, Deramaxx, and Galliprant. Choice is often based on availability, cost, and presence of other systemic diseases. Galliprant is a good choice for any dogs with liver or kidney enzyme elevations.
   iii. For owners resistant to its use, here is an example conversation on how we recommend its usage:
      1. *"Based on how you describe Fluffy's mobility at home, paired with my exam findings today, I do feel this is all due to arthritis. I can tell by feeling her knees and elbows that she has degenerative changes with muscle loss and thickened joints. There comes a time where we need to weigh comfort with side effects. Though these medications can cause side effects like GI upset and kidney/liver changes, they also have great benefits to where Fluffy feels better and is able to do the things she loves again. If you are open to it, why don't we try a 2 week trial with Rimadyl, and see how Fluffy does on it. If you can tell she feels better, I would continue it long term. We recommend blood work every 6-12 months in order to stay on top of her health while on this medication."*

Dr. Gabby Tip on NSAID use

Be sure to get baseline bloodwork and repeat a few weeks later. Always need to consider GI effects, many dogs do not show GI signs yet the NSAID is affecting their GIT. Galliprant is targeted for OA specifically. Clinically I have some dogs that do not get the pain relief from this medication as they do from traditional NSAIDs.

Tips:

Minimizing complications associated with NSAIDs:

- No concurrent glucocorticoids and use a washout period between steroids and NSAIDs or vice versa (also a washout when switching between NSAIDs)
- Baseline and routine screening CBC and chemistry and UA panel in all, not just older patients
- Maintain hydration and give with food
- Just because a dog does not respond to one NSAID it does not mean that they will not benefit from another.
- Very well studied class of drugs in dogs and use veterinary specific only.
- NO ASPIRIN!!! Vets and owners should be aware and specifically ask if the owner is giving anything OTC.

Hillier, T. N., Watt, M. M., Grimes, J. A., Berg, A. N., Heinz, J. A., & Dickerson, V. M. (2025). Dogs receiving cyclooxygenase-2-sparing nonsteroidal anti-inflammatory drugs and/or nonphysiologic steroids are at risk of severe gastrointestinal ulceration. Journal of the American Veterinary Medical Association, 263(3), 1-8. Retrieved Nov 21, 2025, from https://doi.org/10.2460/javma.24.06.0430

Lascelles BD, McFarland JM, Swann H. Guidelines for safe and effective use of NSAIDs in dogs. Vet Ther. 2005 Fall;6(3):237-51. PMID: 16299670.

h. **Amantadine:**

   i. This is a drug with many mechanisms of action. In human medicine, it has been used as an antiviral. How it works to treat chronic pain is through antagonizing NMDA receptors in the central nervous system, which is similar to how ketamine works. It also helps neuropathic pain.

   ii. You should consider its use as a second or third medication added to the dog's regimen because gabapentin and NSAIDs will always be your best first choices. It is a great add on when your patient has worsening chronic pain, and it has been shown to complement NSAIDs well when you find an NSAID alone is not helping a patient's comfort.

   iii. There are no known side effects with this drug.

   - **Dr. Gabby Tip:** GI side effects can occur especially in dogs with GI disease, such as IBD. I have had a few IBD dogs do ok where we start at a low dose. Can cause agitation (I have seen this once in practice). Some dogs may drink more due to dry mouth. Can be SID or BID, many dogs do better with BID. Careful with renal/hepatic, cardiac patients.

Quick doses of our favorite drugs:

- **Adequan:**
  - It comes in a 5 mL (100 mg/ml) vial, and you often sell it by the vial.
  - Dose 0.02 mL/lb (1 ml per 50 lbs).
  - With either protocol mentioned below, Adequan can be discontinued after 6+ months if the owner does not feel it is helping anymore. It can always be restarted at a later date again with the protocols mentioned below if symptoms flare..
  - Dosing schedule varies, we use one of the two protocols:
    - 4.4 mg/kg IM or SQ twice weekly for 4 weeks, then once weekly for 2 weeks, then once every 3-4 weeks long term.
    - 4.4 mg/kg IM or SQ twice weekly for 4 weeks, then once monthly long term.

- **Amantadine:** 3-5 mg/kg PO SID
  - Always use with other medications.
  - Data from studies indicate that BID dosing may be more effective in dogs and cats.

- **Gabapentin:** 5-20 mg/kg PO BID
  - Start with a lower dosage at SID to BID, then build. You can increase to TID over time. Building will help to decrease sedative side effects.
  - **Dr. Gabby Tip:** When possible, I aim for TID due to pharmacokinetics. I have clients start at bedtime for 2-3 days, then go to BID, and then see if they can get to a more steady state TID (not always possible due to owner schedules).

- **Galliprant (grapiprant):** 2 mg/kg PO SID
  - Best given on an empty stomach an hour before feeding.

- **Rimadyl (carprofen):** 4.4 mg/kg PO SID (or 2.2 mg/kg PO BID)
  - Give with food to prevent GI upset.

Basic plans based on age

Pre-arthritis (middle age to early senior): Dogs with no clinical signs or minimal historical signs Many puppies have been dx with OA. Puppies should be evaluated (orthopedic and neuro exam) especially in dogs with family history (when this information is available), or if a predisposed breed..

- Ensure they are maintaining lean body weight as well as an appropriate exercise routine.
- Recommend a daily joint supplement, by prepping owners for the idea that even at this age, there are already degenerative changes starting to occur. Our favorite to begin with is an omega 3 fatty acid. See above for options.
- Go over some of the signs an owner may see develop over time so that they can start actively monitoring their pet.

Dogs with mild to moderate signs of arthritis: These dogs can be any age, though typically they are older adults or seniors.

- Consider a prescription joint diet.
    - This is the easiest way to get their dog the needed amount of omega 3's, so there is no need for additional supplementation.
- Continue daily joint supplements (Omegas, PSGAGs, UC-II, GLM) and you may want to add additional options.
    - If your owner started an omega 3, then you can ask them to add in glucosamine +/- Adequan.
- NSAIDs. Generally a first-line analgesic for the management of canine OA pain
    - Next, you can add in an NSAID of your choice. You can start a 10-14 day trial, and then follow up with the owner to see if they noticed any effect. Trials for 3-4 weeks are often warranted.

- If so, tell them to use it as needed when their pet seems "slower than normal." However, the owner should tell you if they feel their pet may benefit from daily use over time. There may become a point where an NSAID is beneficial on a routine basis.

- **Dr. Gabby Tip:** If recommending NSAIDs on an "as needed" basis, it is important to remember that these medications often need to be given consistently to achieve an effective analgesic effect. Many owners may not fully understand what "as needed" means, so it is essential to provide specific guidelines, such as: "Give the medication when you notice [specific sign or behavior] and continue for [specific duration]." Clear instructions help ensure safe and effective use.

- Gabapentin trial.
    - Initially, we will start a pet on gabapentin every 12-24 hours. You can start a 10-14 day trial, and then follow up with the owner to see if they noticed any effect. Dr. Gabby notes that some dogs need to be on it for a month or longer to see benefits. Also make sure to be dosing appropriately and don't be afraid to increase the dose if they are not drowsy but you still have signs of pain.
    - The KEY is letting the owner know the effect will be mild. They may notice their dog is following them around more or seems to get up the stairs more easily. The goal is to find a dose that will control pain but also not make them extremely lethargic. Have the owner call if their dog seems too sedate and out of their normal routine.

- Alternative modalities.
    - Physical therapy can be very helpful here in helping dogs to maintain lean muscle mass through a combination of an underwater treadmill, balance exercises, etc.
    - **Dr. Gabby Tip:** Mention multi-modal approach and evidence based modalities that have been used to manage pain, such as photobiomodulation (Laser), PEMF, shockwave therapy and of course manual therapy!! Manual therapy is crucial in my opinion and very underutilized!

- Environmental support needs to be started here, if not already implemented. This is very important!
    - Mention tips that make the home mobility friendly with non-slip rugs, orthopedic beds, preventing their dog from climbing stairs unnecessarily, moving food/ water to easily accessible spots, toe grips, etc.

Dogs with moderate to severe mobility issues:

Do the above recommendations, in addition to...

- Daily use of NSAIDs.
    - This drug is an important part of comfort for an arthritic pet, but you MUST ensure your client understands the risks, monitoring parameters (i.e. give with food, discontinue if any inappetance/lethargy/vomiting/diarrhea is noted, etc.), and that they are willing to be diligent and come in for bloodwork every 4-6 months depending on the case (annual is the minimum requirement for those owners who are cost conscious).
    - Just ensure you are on the same page as your owner. Quality of life is a very important factor with these patients.
        - **Example:** 10 year old FS Labrador that struggles to get up easily and go on her regular walks without her Rimadyl. She should have it every day because it improves her quality of life, so long as the owners are ok with the risks.

Dr. Gabby Tip

We are advocating for our patient but the owners know their dog best. This is a family member to them so we must be respectful and try to treat them based on their philosophy of care when possible. It is not our job to judge and withhold care because we do not know about alternative options. Let's educate ourselves and our clients!

I like to bring up QoL scales with clients in a way that is not threatening. An example is: "Have you taken a quality of life scale? These can be a good way to get some information on what aspects of "Kirby's" life we are doing well in and what can use some improvement, we can use it as a guide to get information on what we need to focus on and what we are doing well with" or something like this, otherwise clients can get defensive and upset.

- Add in Adequan injections.
    - Anecdotally, we have many pets that do really well with this medication. Some owners will not start it initially due to cost, so it is always good to recommend one last time at this stage.
    - Cost can be an issue for larger dogs, but we always let owners know that if they can push through the first 6 weeks, it will become a lot more affordable. (See above box for dose and schedule options.)
    - **Dr. Gabby Tip:** Remember that the molecule resembles heparin and so should be d/c prior to surgery or dentals that may require extractions, to minimize bleeding risk. ALSO, I tell people that just because they do not see improvement does not mean that it is not working, it is not a "pain medication". We also need to start this sooner than later, the joint needs some cartilage for it to work.
- Alternative modalities.
    - Consider acupuncture, laser therapy, intra-articular therapies (joint injections) with a variety of products, including orthobiologics, etc.

- Harness or sling support.
    - These are both useful in helping dogs get up from lying down. The Help 'em up harness is one of our favorite brands because it can be left on the patient and has a few handles to help support both the front and hind end. Guiding the dog up and supporting them as they start to walk will help their mobility by loosening up their joints as they walk. It can also be used to support them on stairs to outside.

Dogs with arthritis and kidney disease or other systemic disease:

- For these patients, we try to come up with a multimodal plan that steers away from NSAIDs and leans more into the other drugs, supplements, and alternative therapies like omega 3's, gabapentin, Adequan, acupuncture, etc.
- Galliprant is acceptable for some dogs with bad arthritis and mild/moderate kidney disease or liver value elevations. Use on a case by case basis. We have both used this drug in these patients and not seen significant changes over time. Performing blood work on these patients every 6 months will be helpful in ensuring there are no significant changes, warranting a medication change.

Dr. Gabby Insight on Nerve growth factor (NGF)

Bedinvetmab (Librela; Zoetis) has been used in cases where it may not be appropriate and is currently getting a lot of press for the adverse events being reported. Patient screening is key and it is not for every pain case.

It is labeled for OA without concurrent neurological disease and should be used cautiously with any co-morbidities. At this time in vet med, I have seen a lot of dogs receive this injection that should not have.

I advise blood work, radiographs, and careful patient screening. This is not a benign treatment. In dogs that have OA without concurrent disease or conditions that can exclude them from use it can be a beneficial treatment. However I would NOT say (personally) that it is a first line treatment and that long term use is fine.

I have open and honest conversations with clients (many clients are afraid of using this). Do a pros and cons list and watch for any changes, good or bad, and if the dog has an adverse effect please report it to the company!

References:

- Cachexia and Sarcopenia: Emerging Syndromes of Importance in Dogs and Cats. L.M. Freeman: J Vet Intern Med 2012;26:3-1
- Comparative therapeutic efficacy and safety of type-II collagen (uc-II), glucosamine and chondroitin in arthritic dogs: pain evaluation by ground force plate. R C Gupta 1, T D Canerdy, J Lindley, M Konemann, J Minniear, B A Carroll, C Hendrick, J T Goad, K Rohde, R Doss, M Bagchi, D Bagch. J Anim Physiol Anim Nutr (Berl). October 2012;96(5):770-7.
- Lascelles BD, Gaynor JS, Smith ES, Roe SC, Marcellin-Little DJ, Davidson G, Boland E, Carr J. Amantadine in a multimodal analgesic regimen for alleviation of refractory osteoarthritis pain in dogs. J Vet Intern Med. 2008 Jan-Feb;22(1):53-9. doi: 10.1111/j.1939-1676.2007.0014.x. PMID: 18289289.

NOTES:

NOTES:

Otitis Externa in Dogs

Reviewed by Dr. Jeff Tinsley, DVM, DACVD

Common underlying causes of otitis externa

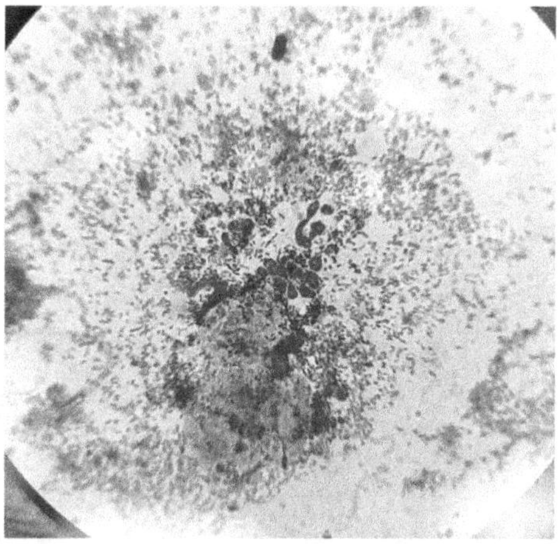

Otitis can be defined literally as inflammation of the ear canal. There is always a reason for the otitis, and they very often come with a secondary infection that requires treatment in addition to addressing the underlying causes. If no infection is present (based on cytology), then we can focus on controlling underlying factors from which the inflammation was derived.

Otitis externa can be broken down in four broad categories. Here is a non-exhaustive list of factors you will encounter in practice:

- **Primary factors:**
  - Management (or elimination) of these factors controls the root cause of the problem.
  - Examples: ALLERGY!!, Otodectes mites, growths (masses, polyps), foreign bodies, endocrine disease (hypothyroidism, etc.)

- **Secondary factors:**
  - Treating these will provide temporary relief. All other factors must be addressed to prevent recurrence.
  - Examples: Bacteria, yeast, overcleaning, medication reactions

- **Perpetuating factors:**
  - These occur due to changes in the anatomy and physiology of the ear in response to chronic otitis. These are not primary triggers, but exacerbate otitis externa.
  - Examples: mineralization/calcification, otitis media/interna

- **Predisposing factors:**
  - These factors increase the *risk* of development of otitis, but do NOT trigger otitis outright.
  - Examples: Swimming (excessive moisture), excessive fur growth in canals, poor ear confirmation (think naturally stenotic/small canals of Frenchies and other brachycephalics)

Four types of ear infections in dogs (often a combo)

1. Yeast (Malassezia, Candida)
2. Bacteria (cocci- Staph, Strep, Enterococcus)
3. Bacteria (rods- Pseudomonas, Proteus, E. coli)
4. Parasitic (ear mites-less common)

Creating a smooth otic appointment summary

1. Diagnose if there is infection present and type of infection through ear cytology +/- ear smear for mites.

2. Examine your patient and check ears last because they are most painful.

3. Clean the ear with saline if the patient allows and if you are unable to see due to significant debris. You want to visualize the tympanic membrane.

4. Determine what underlying causes to address today.

5. Discuss your treatment plan.

Creating smooth otic appointments - Our approach

Understanding this basic approach to ear inflammation and subsequent secondary infections will help you succeed in the majority of your otitis appointments. Be sure to master the communication points, which will help you avoid frustrated owners. For 'frustrating cases' (because they do happen), see our last section.

1. **Diagnosis of infection:** If the patient allows, have your tech get ear swabs right away and start running the cytology for you before you enter the room. This saves you time and can allow you to start mentally preparing treatment options based on the type of infection and the exam findings (i.e. is the eardrum intact?, etc.). However, if the ear canals have a large volume of cerumen (ear wax) visibly present. Be mindful that you may want to examine the ears prior to sampling as the wax can be pushed *deeper* into the canal and occlude your vision on otoscopic exam.

2. **Examine the pet:** Next, we enter the room to perform the exam on our patient. We recommend examining the patient's ears last due to the discomfort associated with the infection, as this decreases the patient's stress level. Dr. Jeff recommends that if one ear is less affected, begin with the better ear to get the patient used to otic examination.

    a. During our exam, we will not be discussing everything we see in detail unless something surprises us, as we are really here today to focus on the ears. While performing the exam, we will tell the owner this...

    b. *"I'm going to do a full exam first to be thorough, and then we're going to focus on Fluffy's ears. They can be painful to examine so waiting until the end will allow us to assess him from head to toe today." (Shows the value of the visit and gives you something to say while you are focusing)*

        i. Keep in mind that other dermatologic findings like paw irritation, brown fur staining (from saliva) or skin lesions may increase your suspicion of underlying causes like allergies and prompt additional questions to the client.

When we perform our otic exam, we are assessing the entire external canal along with the eardrum to ensure it is intact. You should assess for erythema, excess cerumen, stenosis, etc. *Tip from Dr. Jeff:* You should also palpate the canals externally to assess for pliability (are the soft? fibrotic/scarred? Hard like a rock/mineralized?). It is also important to look for other abnormalities that may lead to an infection (see factors at beginning of the chapter). Sometimes, you need to clean the ear out in order to look for these things if there is significant ear debris.

3. Clean the pet's ears, as allowed: **This tip removes debris to set the pet up for successful treatment as well as allows you time outside of the exam room** to start thinking about causes and your plan. As a new vet, you can also use this time to consult with another doctor before discussing your plan with the owner.

    a. **Tip from Dr. Jeff:** Plain saline is a good option for cleaning as many ear cleaners can occlude your vision with bubbles.

    b. *"Oh no! That ear looks very painful. Ok, let me start by cleaning the ear to see if he will allow me to look in there a little better. I am going to take Louis to the treatment area where we have all of our supplies to give him a thorough cleaning. We will be right back."*

4. Determine which underlying factors need to be addressed today:

    a. **First time offenders:** With your first time or infrequent offenders, keep it simple.
        i. *"Louis had a bacteria and yeast infection that we will treat with these ear drops and this cleaner today. Since this is his first infection, we'll see how he responds and recommend a recheck to make sure it's resolved. All ear infections have an underlying cause. Allergies are the most common. To prepare you, IF this infection is persistent or if he has a second infection this year, then I may recommend a diet trial as a next step."*
        ii. If you have a very motivated client and extra time before your next appointment, it is certainly appropriate to begin a strict 8 week Rx elimination diet trial on day one (see pruritus and allergy chapter for diet trial specifics).

    b. **Recurrent otitis externa patients:** With patients that have recurrent ear infections within a year, we start having a more serious conversation around causes and start setting up expectations for owners as to next recommended steps. Always make sure these pets are on their flea and tick prevention (isoxazolines preferred). Our client communication on recurrent otitis externa patients may go like this:
        i. Discuss the cause: *"The most common cause of infection in both ears is allergies. I also sometimes see mites and other conditions occurring. Smaller ear canals or excessive fur in some breeds can also lead to chronic ear disease*

(think Cocker Spaniel with heavy ears). We also sometimes have to address middle ear infections and even tumors in older patients."

ii. **Focus the owner on the immediate hurdle of getting rid of the infection AND controlling inflammation:** *"But right now, the ear is so swollen and painful that I cannot get a great look in the ear. So, what I'd like to focus on for this visit is addressing the infection and reducing inflammation."*

iii. **Set expectation of needing a recheck:** *"He will definitely need to come back and see me in two weeks, so we can assess improvement and hopefully at that time I can get a better look when he is less painful. I want you to come back even if you think the ear infection has resolved because they often look better, but the ears can still have bacteria or yeast present that we need to continue treating."*

iv. **Set expectations of reassessing otitis and creating a long term plan at recheck:** *"Based on response to therapy, we will discuss how to prevent ear infections at the next visit. This may mean he needs to be on allergy medications seasonally or long term, consider a prescription diet trial\ to rule out a food allergy, get routine ear cleanings.. Patients with recurrent ear infections always have an underlying cause that we need to address. He may still get infections on and off, but the goal is to give you tips at home that will help reduce their frequency in the future. Some pets that have recurrent ear infections like Louis, ultimately need to see a dermatologist which we can discuss further at our recheck."*

v. **Discuss your treatment plan.** We always ask owners if they think they can get ear medications into their pet at home to help guide us on what type of plan (leave in or not) will help set the pet and owner up for compliance and success.

    1. **Pro tip from Dr. Jeff:** You may also ask your vet tech to show them how to apply meds to increase their confidence and allow you to be more efficient and get into your next room.

Client communication summary for recurrent otitis externa patients

- Discuss the suspected underlying factors.
- Focus the owner on the immediate goal of controlling inflammation and getting rid of any secondary infection.
- Set expectations of needing a recheck.
- Set expectations of reassessing otitis (to ensure inflammation is controlled and infection is resolved) and creating a long term plan at the recheck (i.e. elimination diet trial, etc.).

Otitis externa treatment options

Mild to moderate otitis can be treated for 7-10 days with more severe infections for 14+ days based on your recheck. The key is to appropriately treat infection, confirm infection has cytologically resolved and ensure you are addressing the underlying cause. This highlights how critical rechecks are so you can assess these factors! We have included some ear medications below that we commonly use in practice. Many are commercial products, and others are compounded medications you can make in-house or at a local compounding pharmacy. **Do not forget about systemic anti-inflammatories such as Apoquel, steroids, the newer Zenrelia or sometimes cyclosporine (Atopica) that may be needed. See the treatments for pruritus in the pruritus and allergy chapter for more information on these medications.** We use anti-inflammatories in cases where pets show some discomfort,are exhibiting incessant head shaking/scratching or have excessive erythema on otic exam. Very mild cases may respond to Apoquel, but cases of severe erythema benefit more from temporary steroid use. They can make your patients considerably more comfortable, especially until the ear medication starts kicking in. Dr. Jeff wanted to remind you that Atopica is the exception because it may take 1 month to *begin* reducing inflammation.

Ear medication thoughts from Dr. Jeff

- **Medication Disclaimer**: Be mindful of the class of each drug you are using in your ear meds. Be intentional when you are making choices for your infections.
  - **Example:**
    - If a patient has recurrent cocci and the volume is not improving at recheck (based on cytology), you may consider switching classes of antibiotics or performing ear culture/sensitivity.
    - If a patient has extreme ear inflammation, consider switching to an ear formulation with a more potent steroid or adding an oral steroid.
    - In some cases, your ear antimicrobial is working, but excess cerumen and discharge is so great, switching to a better ceruminolytic cleaner is the right choice.
  - **His tips:**
    - The more you use ear meds and pay attention to what you are using, the more this will become second nature.
    - In addition, regular topical applications at home are preferred if the owner is able to treat the ears. This gives you more control over dosing.
    - Ears that have excess ear wax may inactivate your antimicrobials. In which case, very "gunky" productive ears may never resolve with leave-in options as they may require regular cleansing prior to placement of antimicrobial ointments.

- **Yeast infection alone:** Treatment options for a straightforward infection include Miconazole/DexSP, Surolan, Tresaderm, Easotic, or DuOtic if a leave-in is needed (new drug as of 2025).

- **Bacterial infection (cocci) with or without yeast:** Treatment options for a straightforward infection include Easotic, Surolan, Tresaderm, and if a leave-in is needed: Claro, Osurnia)
  - **Side note:** Dosing of ear medications can be tricky for owners (put 'xx number of drops'' or 'a small squeeze" into the ear). Pay attention to this when assessing ear medications on the market to stock ones that are easier to dose.
    - **Example:** Easotic features a pump design on top where 1 mL equals a single pump vs. other drugs have a nozzle that requires owner to dose (drops)

- **Bacterial infection (rods +/- cocci) with or without yeast:** Treatment options for a straightforward or complicated infection include Posatex (more specific to rods than cocci), Mometamax (can get some rods), Keto-Triz ear cleaner + large animal Baytril + DexSP (safer option, see formula we use below).
  - **Note:** Rod based infections can be unpredictable. Some clinicians consider ear culture/sensitivity and adjust therapy based on results.

- **Suspect Resistant ear infection:** Often, you will see minimal response at your recheck in resistance cases. Consider an ear culture and sensitivity of the ear and be familiar with common contaminants that can grow. Consider adjustment to a more broad spectrum (Baytril) medication like Keto-Triz ear cleaner + large animal Baytril + DexSP and/or Triz EDTA + SSD cream. These are very difficult cases, and Dr. Jeff wanted to reiterate that it is often best to involve a dermatologist at this point.

Ear cultures/sensitivities: challenges and options

By: Dr. Jeff

- These are somewhat controversial.
- According to *Small Animal Dermatology,* resistance to a particular antibiotic in vitro may not correlate with clinical response because direct application of medication to the ear canal results in higher antibiotic concentration than with systemic medication.
- In practice, this means that an antibiotic susceptibility result for an antibiotic like enrofloxacin, may read as "resistant", but this does not necessarily reflect the much higher strength of the concentration of that antibiotic if it were applied topically.
- Therefore, ear cultures are best reserved for cases of otitis media to guide systemic antibiotic therapy. Unfortunately, cultures of the middle ear are challenging to collect. Middle ear cultures are collected best under full anesthesia via video otoscopy (often at a referral center). Some studies have indicated that middle ear cultures do not always reflect the same susceptibility profile of the external canal organisms.

So what do we do in the real world??

- In chronic otitis externa cases, referral is the best option, especially if you suspect concurrent otitis media as a perpetuating factor.
- Have a clear discussion with your client. If the client expresses that this will never be a financial option, then it is reasonable to consider ear culture/sensitivity from the external canal and treat as best you can from those results.
    - You can consider an antibiotic in these cases. Start with 1 month of therapy, but note that most cases require extended antibiotic courses (2-3 months). Treating 1 month past clinical resolution may be warranted. In addition, be sure to adjust your topical treatments based on the culture if possible, but keep in mind that your topical antibiotic choice could still be effective based on topical application regardless of the in vitro results. Adjusting your topical cleanser (disinfectant vs. ceruminolytic) and choosing a good systemic anti-inflammatory should also be considered based on case severity.

- **Ruptured tympanic membrane/Ototoxicity (Tips from Dr. Jeff):**
  - The exact prevalence of ototoxicity is not known. Some studies indicate that Triz EDTA was shown to not be ototoxic. Aminoglycosides (gentamicin, amikacin, etc.) have been more commonly implicated at risk of ototoxicity.
  - Technically, there is no 100% safe medication that can be applied to the ear canal with no risks of side effects. And unfortunately, oral antibiotics may not treat otitis externa well, so it is recommended to reserve their use for otitis interna/ media cases.
  - Appropriate systemic options ("So what do we do in the real world") are warranted. You can also consider gabapentin for pain. Since most of pain from otitis is related to inflammation, most dermatologists reach for steroids (consider prednisone starting at 1 mg/kg/day and taper) pending bloodwork monitoring.
  - Treat for 3-4 weeks and recheck, as some dogs require treatment for up to 6-8 weeks. The tympanic membrane may take several months to regrow.
  - Topical therapy: Discuss this in detail and risks with the owner. Saline or Tris EDTA may be safer options, but are not always effective at clearing infection.
  - In these cases, consider medications that tend to be 'safer' for the middle ears of most dogs which include miconazole, enrofloxacin, dexamethasone, and Tris-EDTA. A frank and documented discussion with owners is important here as there is no guarantee that these are safe so they have to understand there is some risk. Some pet's eardrums may not heal or may continue to have recurrent ear infections that are nonresponsive to your treatment plan. In these cases the patients need to be referred to a dermatologist to have the middle/inner ear flushed under general anesthesia (video otoscopy).

Notes about the above ear medications

- ***Mometamax:** We have seen a few dogs (all small breed dogs with visually intact eardrums) lose hearing on this medication (including Monica's dog, a Westie named Frodo). Note from Dr. Jeff: a visually intact ear drum may have microtears that are not evident on otic evaluation. In all cases, the hearing came back over time. So when we prescribe this medication, we warn owners that in really rare cases we have seen hearing loss. So, if they notice deafness, they should stop the drops right away and call the hospital. Again, this is one of our go-to medications, and this phenomenon is super rare, but just something to be aware of. Dr. Jeff recommends immediate flushing of the ears with saline in these cases (best done in the clinic, if possible).

Ear recipes from Dr. Ashley and Dr. Monica:

- **Miconazole 1% with DexSP:** This is a mixture you can make in-house. You create it by removing 6 mL from Miconazole and adding in 6 mL of injectable DexSP (4mg/ml).
- **Keto-Triz ear cleaner + large animal Baytril + DexSP:** Remove 19 mL of Keto-Triz cleaner from bottle. Add 20 mL of large animal Baytril (100 mg/mL), and then add 6 mL of DexSP. Have the owner instill 0.5 mL into the ear canal once daily for 10-14 days.
- **Triz EDTA + SSD cream**: Add 50 grams of 1% SSD cream to a 12 ounce bottle of Triz EDTA. Have the owner instill 1 mL into the ear canal once daily for 10-14 days.

Pro tip from Dr. Jeff

Avoidance of all lanolin products is highly recommended. Lanolin is a waxy compound that some leave-in compounded products are mixed with for otic application. It is extremely difficult to flush and remove this product in patients who have an adverse reaction to the lanolin.

Tips to know when managing otitis externa:

- **Always get ear swab samples before cleaning.** If possible, have your assistant get samples when they are checking the pet in (only if they can do so safely alone). They can start this while you finish up your last appointment. Often our cytologies are done before we have even seen the dog, which helps you to save time and stay efficient!

- **Clean the yucky ears out, as this usually helps you get a better view.** Saline is a great first choice ear cleaner because it is safe in a ruptured eardrum and does not cause pain in a sensitive ear (as compared to other alcohol based cleaners).

- **With some painful patients, you may only get 'one shot' to look in the ear.** So if appropriate, have the ears cleaned out first. If the dog is too painful for you to perform your otic exam, you have three options.

    - **First option** is to offer to sedate their pet. Sedation can be nice because you are able to clean the ear thoroughly and remove any occluding hair with minimal stress or pain to your patient. You can then easily examine the ear prior to reversing sedation.

- **Tips from Dr. Jeff:**
    - Be very mindful that if the ear drum is ruptured, ear flushing of a sedated patient can cause fluid to flow through the eustachian tube connecting to an unprotected trachea. This is an aspiration risk. Flushing (unless under full anesthesia with an E-tube) should be done with extreme caution.
    - Minor ear cleaning should be otherwise safe. Consider having the patient on a tilted surface to prevent excess fluid going where we don't want it to go.

- **Second option** is to consider sending the dog home with medications and then have them come back in a few days once the inflammation has subsided. This is a great option if you are concerned there may be a more serious infection present or a ruptured eardrum.
    - Start your patient on a short prednisone course (5-7 days) +/- KetoTriz ear cleaner and recheck in 5-7 days. Consider gabapentin +/- trazodone combination to give prior to the recheck if you think the dog will benefit from it to allow you to finish your exam. This combination allows you to get a second exam in, so you can finalize your treatment plan of topical medications, etc.

- **Third option** is to consider treating the ear ONLY if you feel comfortable doing so, but warn owners of possible adverse side effects if there were to be a damaged eardrum (ototoxicity, vestibular signs, etc.). If these adverse side effects occur, owners get very upset if they are not warned about them.

- **Have your tech show the owner how to clean the ear and go over how to medicate the ear** if you are not doing a leave-in treatment. You will be surprised how many owners have no idea how to clean their dog's ears or are performing it wrong at home. You can even have a bookmarked Youtube video to email them!

- **You should always send each owner home with an ear cleaner.** Cleaning the ears is one of the best ways to prevent an infection when they are dirty or after any water exposure (bathing, swimming), and most ear ointments will not work until excess cerumen has been removed prior to treatment.

- **If you have a pet that is INCESSANTLY shaking their head, be warned that an aural hematoma can occur.** We will do one of two things depending on how concerned we are about this complication. Most of the time, we will send these dogs home on prednisone to go along with their ear medications, and this is sufficient in preventing a hematoma. However, there have been certain instances where the pet was SO incessant with their ear flapping in the clinic (especially after it was cleaned) that we went ahead and gave them an injection of DexSP before sending home with prednisone to start the next day. Always ask the owner before doing this, but this method allows us to ensure the flapping stops quickly. The few times we have done this were situations where the dog came in with a very painful, inflamed ear due to shaking their head for a long time. After the cleaning in the hospital, the dog continued audibly flapping incessantly. Giving DexSP helps the dog feel better quicker, and many owners are thankful. For a dog that has a minimally inflamed ear, we will prescribe Apoquel instead.

The frustrating otitis cases

Sometimes we get here, and that's ok. What will help you succeed is clear communication of expectations and a plan. With recurrent or difficult to treat ear infections, you must keep the list of possible factors (as noted at the top of the chapter) in mind. It can be very frustrating to an owner when they feel that we cannot keep their pet free of otitis flares. One of the main reasons a client sees a new vet is when they feel their pet's condition is not resolving or being managed appropriately. Setting client expectations is key here.

Be open and up front with them from the start. Explain that otitis can be frustrating and require multiple therapies to prevent in the future. We tell clients that our goal is to decrease the frequency of ear flares , so they understand their pet may still flare intermittently. By utilizing all of our tips above and treating for any of these additional causes, you will get better client satisfaction and patient happiness.

If we have an ear infection that is difficult to get under control despite taking all the appropriate precautions, we will consider referral to a dermatologist. If that is not possible due to cost, then consider ear culture and a sedated deep flush (under full anesthesia preferred for safety). Start having this conversation early, once you notice the patient is becoming refractory to treatment or having recurrent infections. Owners can warm up to the idea over time.

To pluck or not to pluck?

Insight by Dr. Jeff

In some cases of recurrent otitis, extreme amounts of fur can perpetuate inflammation and physically prevent medication from reaching the ear canal walls (not unlike a foreign body). You can consider sedated fur removal for these cases. Be aware that some cases can flare from the physical trauma of fur removal. Avoid removal of ALL fur and remove enough that medications should be able move freely through the fur.

If needed, 3-5 days of a steroid like prednisone at 1 mg/kg/day can keep the ears more comfortable. If otic flares continue or worsen despite fur plucking, they shouldn't be continued. If patients feel great relief post plucking, they can be continued as needed every 2-3 months. Be sure to control the underlying cause of the otitis as well. Excess fur growth on its own is considered a predisposing factor of otitis, but not a primary one.

References:

- Muller, George H., et al. Muller & Kirk's Small Animal Dermatology. 7th ed., Elsevier, 2013.
- Woodward, Michelle. "Otitis Media and Interna in Animals - Ear Disorders." Merck Veterinary Manual, Merck & Co., Inc., 2020
- Clegg J., Souza C., Brame B.; Tolerability of Otic Solutions Containing Different Enrofloxacin Concentrations in Dogs with Healthy Ears. J Am
- Anim Hosp Assoc 1 September 2023; 59 (5): 214–218. doi: https://doi.org/10.5326/JAAHA-MS-7363
- Gotthelf LN. Diagnosis and treatment of otitis media in dogs and cats. Vet Clin North Am Small Anim Pract 2004;34:469–87
- FDA approves treatment for yeast ear infections in dogs. U.S. Food and Drug Administration. March 15, 2024. Accessed June 24, 2025. https://www.fda.gov/animal-veterinary/cvm-updates/fda-approvestreatment-yeast-ear-infections-dogs
- Miller, Julia. "What's New in Otitis Externa Treatment Options." Today's Veterinary Practice, 2025, todaysveterinarypractice.com/pharmacology/whats-new-in-otitis-externa-treatment-options/.

NOTES:

NOTES:

Pruritus and Allergies in dogs

Reviewed by Dr. Jeff Tinsley, DVM, DACVD

Pruritic dogs are one of THE most common cases you will see in general practice. Allergies make up a large percentage of these cases and that will be what we focus on in this chapter. These cases will be really frustrating to owners who do not understand quick fixes are not always possible. Many clients will also struggle to understand the value of rechecks when their dog looks better, yet rechecks are the key to ensuring appropriate treatment and reduction of chronic skin issues. Setting expectations with the owner and providing thorough communication will be of the utmost importance in reducing owner confusion and frustration. Let's start with a quick review of the basic clinical signs of allergies in dogs before we dig into our approach and client communication tips.

Common presentations for allergies

- **Paw licking:** This is often the most common clinical sign of pruritus noticed noticed by owners at these appointments. Be sure to check each paw's dorsal and palmar/plantar interdigital space, each nail, paw pad, etc. to be thorough. Be sure to notate which paws are affected, so you can revisit these specific areas at your recheck to assess for improvement.
    - The most common cause of paw licking is pruritus due to allergies, though other causes such as secondary bacterial or yeast infection, anxiety, boredom, pain, foreign bodies, ectoparasites (Demodex), cutaneous drug reaction, trauma, and more can cause it too. If you are not seeing any improvement with your treatment plan, these are other differentials to consider at the recheck. Note from Dr. Jeff: Behavioral dermatoses are rare and typically do not present as licking of multiple paws, which is a common allergic presentation.

- **Ear flapping/shaking with or without an ear infection:** See our chapter on otitis externa for thorough notes on this clinical sign.

- **Pruritus that precedes skin lesions:** You may see a healthy coat or notice changes consistent with dermatitis (see below). Almost all cases of allergy began with grossly normal skin with pruritus leading to lesions and secondary infections.
    - **Pro tip from Dr. Jeff:** Always ask if the owners noticed lesions first or itching/licking first. If they aren't sure, you can do an itch relief trial with anti-pruritics for two weeks and have them monitor for what comes first when the medications are stopped.

- **Salivary staining on paws or focal areas (often brown fur)**

- **Dermatitis:** You may only have one clinical sign or a combination such as erythema, papules, pustules, lichenification, hyperpigmentation, seborrhea, excoriations, or more. In dogs with true allergies, these are almost always secondary to pruritus/self-mutilation.

- **Moth eaten or diffuse alopecia:** Often evident of a secondary bacterial folliculitis or Malassezia dermatitis. Skin cytology is required to differentiate which is present. Sometimes it's both!

- **Lichenification:** You may see a cobblestone appearance or 'elephant skin,' (check axilla and neck closely!). This is often indicative of chronic self trauma. It is very common to have a concurrent yeast or deep bacterial infection present. Yeast is more common in these cases, but skin cytology is needed for appropriate identification and treatment of the secondary factors.

When it is not allergies

Not every skin condition is due to allergies. Differentials like pemphigus, other autoimmune diseases, metabolic conditions (endocrine disease, hepatocutaneous syndrome), MRSP, and more have tricked us. So, here are a few clues that it may NOT be allergies...

- **Lesions are noticed first.** If the owner is certain the lesions seemed to appear prior to pruritus, begin with a skin cytology for secondary bacterial/yeast infection and rule out differentials such as: ringworm, ectoparasites, endocrine diseases, autoimmune disease, cutaneous neoplasia. For the most part these conditions don't start pruritic with the exception of parasites like fleas or scabies.

- **The dog is not responding to your basic treatment plan.** Make sure drug doses are correct, check owner compliance, and that rechecks are occurring, etc. If the dog worsens despite good ectoparasite prevention (ideally an isoxazoline), appropriate treatment, consider repeat cytology, cultures, biopsy, referral, etc.

- **The dog is not feeling well.** Examples include a fever, severe lethargy, or limping because their paw pads are sore. We have seen dogs limp because of a severe infection secondary to allergies, but we have also seen odd paw pad deformities due to allergic reactions to medications, autoimmune conditions , etc. Most cases of allergies feel systemically normal or presentation.

- **People in the home also have lesions.** Think zoonotic diseases like ringworm or scabies.

How to systematically approach an appointment with pruritic symptoms

The approach mentioned below will work for the majority of your pruritic dogs and will help you avoid frustrated clients. Be sure to be thorough, systematic, and document appropriately to make your rechecks run smoothly. Throughout each step, we will discuss important client communication points to bring up to owners to ensure you cover all of your bases.

The end of the chapter will give you specific communication points for certain situations. Be sure to clearly explain underlying causes, what you are treating, set expectations, and stress the importance of rechecks in order to tailor therapy appropriately. **Owners need to understand that if their dog's pruritus is diagnosed as allergies that this is a chronic, non-curable condition. Their dog will now need routine visits in order to make them comfortable and that therapies that once worked may not work later in life.** This occurs because a patient's hypersensitivity to their allergens will often worsen over the years. Recheck exams allow you to work together as a team to keep their dog comfortable. Lastly, it is important owners understand that the goal is to improve symptoms to a manageable state through a combination of the steps mentioned below.

General approach for a straightforward pruritus case

1. **Rule out ectoparasites/flea allergy:** If not on reliable flea prevention, send the owner home with it and multiple doses for future months.
2. **Diagnostics:** Skin cytology +/- other diagnostics to guide treatment plan.
3. **Treatment plan:** Majority of our cases go home with both topical and systemic medications.
4. **Client Communication:** Discuss underlying causes, set expectations, and stress the need for a recheck where you will ensure complete resolution and discuss prevention and management strategies.

STEP 1: Rule out a flea allergy (and mange (scabies or Demodex) if possible):

Your first step is to ALWAYS rule out a flea allergy. EVERY. SINGLE. TIME. Classic distribution continues to be an alopecic appearance at the tail base/hind limb region and hind legs, excoriations, and intense sudden pruritus. Some clinicians describe this as a "Winnie the Pooh" look because the dog looks like it has no pants! You will also see dogs without hair loss too. Some only exhibit pruritus and erythema on the caudal, ventral abdomen. Many clients will swear they do not see a flea on their dog, so here are some tips if you hit a wall here.

- Explain to your client that adult fleas make up less than 5% of the flea population, because they are groomed away by the dog. This can make it very difficult to find a flea on a pet. All it takes is one flea, and a flea allergy is something very easy to treat. *A flea comb can be your best friend in finding a flea!* **It is important owners understand that this step is just part of the process because we have to rule out causes in order to be systematic in our approach. Insist each animal in their home gets on reliable, vet prescribed flea prevention.**

- **If the dog is not on flea prevention, send the client home with a product THAT DAY.** Fortunately, due to the isoxazoline class of drugs (Bravecto, Nexgard, Simparica, and Credelio), we can rule out both flea allergies and scabies by simply putting them on this medication. This class of preventatives will also resolve most cases of Demodex as well. Make sure to stress this product must be continued year-round for best results. We often tell owners that even though it may not be a flea allergy, flea saliva has also been shown to exacerbate the itch of other forms of allergies, so it is important to prevent them at all times to be thorough.

    - **Caution and some perspective from Dr. Jeff:** Some studies have shown correlation with isoxazolines and worsening of seizures due to idiopathic epilepsy. Therefore many clinicians chose a different class of prevention for these cases. If possible, touching base with your nearest neurologist for their opinion is recommended. This is an area of on-going research. Also, most isoxazolines come as chewables. A topical product (like topical Bravecto) may be more appropriate for systemically ill patients.

- **Reminder from Dr. Jeff:** If you suspect an active flea infestation, a discussion of periodic deep cleaning and a client handout is warranted to rid the home of the fleas (see flea allergy dermatitis chapter).

STEP 2: Diagnostics: Skin cytology (EVERY TIME) +/- skin scrape +/- ringworm culture if applicable.

We always start with skin cytology in order to determine what we need to treat (bacteria, yeast, etc.). You may want to do a skin scrape too, if the owner wants to be thorough, and/or you have a suspicion of mites. Perform cytology on the areas that the dog is itching such as the flank, paws, etc.

Pro tip from Dr. Jeff: Avoid the old myth "It smells like yeast." Our noses are not microscopes! Both bacterial and yeast infections can be odorous. Only skin cytology can help us differentiate what we're truly dealing with in the ears.

At the recheck, it is important to perform follow-up cytology, even if it looks healed. Why? Quiet skin can still have a smoldering infection, and if you do not do cytology to ensure the infection is gone, the dog's secondary infection will return within a few days to weeks after treatment ends.

- **Skin cytology**: There are two common methods to choose from, so pick what will get you results based on the appearance of the skin.

    - **Tape prep (easy/our fave):** This method works well on dry lesions. It is best utilized when you do not have overt lesions or moist areas to sample. This is performed by taking a piece of regular, clear scotch tape , and you will press the tape firmly and repeatedly to the lesion/areas of pruritus. Using your Diff-Quick (standard 3 solution set up), skip the fixadent (1st solution) and dip the tape into the red stain (2nd solution) for 5-10 seconds, then into the blue stain (3rd solution) for 5-10 seconds. Gently rinse residual solution off and apply the tape sticky side down onto a microscopic slide.

    - **Impression smear:** This method can be used on any skin lesions. It works best for pustules or moist lesions. It can also be used to get under papules and crusts. To sample, gently, but firmly rub a microscopic slide onto your target skin lesion. Repeat until you can visibly see skin material on the slide. For dryer lesions, start at a 45-degree angle to get under crusts and progress the slide forward decreasing the angle until parallel with the skin. You can sample a pustule by rupturing it with a needle or using the edge of the microscopic slide and the previously mentioned method. For moist or greasy areas, you can gently press the slide directly to the lesion. For claw bed debris, consider collecting with the end of a cotton-tipped swab or a toothpick and rub the sample towards the frosted edge of your slide so it is easy to find.

- **Skin scrape:** This method is utilized for ruling out mites. It is performed by finding an area of hair loss, crusts or pustules and scraping it with a dull 10 blade. For Demodex, you will perform a deep skin scrape until you see a small amount of blood as Demodex live at the bottom of hair follicles where blood vessels are present. The best places to find Demodex are on the paws, muzzle and periocularly, but they can be present anywhere For scabies, you will perform a superficial scrape. The best spots to find them are ear margins and lateral elbows, especially in crusted areas. Again, they can be present anywhere. View mites microscopically by applying your sample to a slide with mineral oil and assess it at 4x or 10x. Remember to lower the light and decrease the size of the diaphragm for best results.

    - **Pro tips from Dr. Jeff:**
        - Familiarize yourself with the eggs, larvae, nymphs and even the feces of each type of mite (yes even the poop!), as you may not always see the adult mites.
        - If the lesions are too close to the eyes for comfort, consider plucking hairs with hemostats and viewing under the same specifications as noted above. This is called a trichogram.

- **Ringworm PCR and culture:** If you notice characteristic signs of ringworm (such as focal, circular alopecia bordered by crusting lesions) or lesions on a human, then this is an important test to perform. Note: Unless secondary bacteria or yeast is present, cases of ringworm are rarely pruritic. Never rely on a Wood's lamp alone, as it does not illuminate all species of dermatophytosis, but it is a good screening test for Microsporum canis. A Wood's lamp is shone on lesions in a darkened room and if M. canis is present, the fur may fluoresce "candy apple green".

    - **Note from Dr. Jeff:** Do not be fooled by glowing skin, crust or scale itself because this is commonly a false positive. Only a fluorescent hair follicle is indicative of true ringworm. The gold standard is to perform a ringworm PCR and culture. A PCR will provide you with faster results than a culture to help raise suspicion and guide treatment. You perform this test by plucking the hair and crusts of a lesion and placing the samples in a sterile, empty tube. You can also use a toothbrush to brush the area and send this in a sterile container as well.

STEP 3: Treatment plan:

Here is a general treatment plan to follow for most pruritus cases. You may start with the top four categories initially, and then you can build to other options over time. Have a frank conversation with your owner to understand what their goals are and explain to them that we can adjust the treatment plan over time as symptoms change.

1. **Flea medication:** Always send home with **flea medications** if they are not on a product currently or are not on one that you feel works well in your area. An isoxazoline should be your go-to. (Assure other pets in the home are also on a reliable flea prevention.)

2. **Antimicrobial therapy tips from Dr. Jeff:** Based on your cytology, if bacteria or yeast is present, topical therapy should be included in your plan. Even widespread infections can be resolved with appropriate topical therapies alone! A reasonable 1st line would be using a 2% chlorhexidine/2% miconazole product at least twice weekly. Chlorhexidine products at 3-4% have even been shown to be effective against resistant Staph infections like MRSP. If you feel systemic antibiotics are warranted, cephalexin, cefpodoxime and clindamycin are reasonable 1st choices and are typically prescribed for 3-4 weeks or 1-2 weeks beyond cytological resolution of infection. Ketoconazole or terbinafine are reasonable choices if oral antifungals are warranted for Malassezia with similar courses prescribed as antibiotics.

    ▽ **Pro tip:** Shorter courses of antimicrobials can be used for minor infections such as 14 days, but recheck exam with repeat cytology to confirm resolution of secondary infection is always warranted. In addition, the more topicals the owner can do, the less systemic antimicrobials we often have to use! Many allergic pets also benefit from long-term topical maintenance with medicated bathing, mousses, wipes, etc.

3. **Anti-itch therapy:** Choose appropriate **anti-itch therapy** because this is the main reason the client brought their pet to see you. Your patient needs some relief. Explain to your owner that there are a variety of options here. If the patient has milder symptoms (pruritus scale of 1-3/10 and mild clinical signs), you can ask the owner if they want to start with milder medications first, then build. If the patient has more severe symptoms (pruritus scale of

4-10/10 and/or moderate to severe dermatitis), you will want to use stronger medications, even if just for a few weeks to get your patient under control. **Remind owners that our goal is to decrease the itch level by 50%,** if we get to 2-3/10, then that is even better. It is important to mention to owners that you may need to adjust medications throughout their dog's life because some antipruritics can become ineffective over time (likely due to worsening allergic disease). We also find that some dogs respond better to one medication over another. **Here are some options to consider:**

- ▽ **Topical Anti-itch (1-3/10 on pruritus scale):** **Douxo calm spray** is a great topical option that restores moisture to the skin/coat. However, it does not treat infection. Consider Douxo Pyo Mousse/wipes if there is active infection. Douxo Calm spray can be used as adjunct to an antihistamine for owners wanting to start with a more #natural approach. Gentacalm spray or Neopredef powder are some other options, however, they contain steroids. Any topical steroid is recommended to be used for no more than 2 weeks as overuse can lead to thinning of the skin and they can exacerbate secondary infections with chronic use. **Epsom salt foot soaks** are great for paws, and the dog can get these 1-2 times daily for 5-10 minutes for 7-10 days or as needed when symptoms flare-up.

- ▽ **Antihistamines (1-3/10 on pruritus scale):** These can be good options if the patient is not very itchy or the owner does not wish to use a "stronger medication" initially. Some studies indicate that antihistamines are roughly 5-10% effective at reducing allergic pruritus. Warn clients that they may not work well to manage the itch and that sometimes one works better than another. We like **Benadryl** (diphenhydramine HCl 2.2 mg/kg every 8-12 hours) and **Zyrtec** (cetirizine HCl 01 mg/kg every 24 hours). Ensure they do not choose a product with a pseudoephedrine in it due to toxicity. Note: veterinarians have been sued over this, so it is best to write down the dose for them in a record and CITE the only active ingredient that should be on the bottle. This ensures that they do not use a product that has a 'D' in it a.k.a. NO DECONGESTANT, and ensure you tell the owner this so that they understand it is toxic to pets.

- ▽ **Temaril-P (1-5/10 on pruritus scale):** This is a great combination medication that is an **antihistamine paired with a low-dose steroid**. You will prescribe a short tapering course over 7-14 days to provide immediate relief. We often will use this product initially to get the inflammation down, and then we will have the owner transition to an antihistamine or non-steroid based antipruritic for longer term relief. It can be cost prohibitive for larger dogs, so we usually reach for it in small to medium sized dogs.

- **Prednisone (4-10/10 on pruritus scale):** As you know, **steroids** are our tried and true medication. They will work fast and are very affordable but are not a great long term option. We usually do a tapering course over 7-21 days based on the severity of the patient, starting with 0.5 mg/kg/day. In owners with financial concerns, it can be used at the lowest effective dose that causes the fewest long-term side-effects, so long as you have a very frank and open conversation with the owner about side effects (document this conversation). This should be considered a last resort and additional bloodwork (CBC/CHEM at least 3 times per year) is recommended with this protocol. Some pets have such severe clinical signs that it is better to keep their dog comfortable on a steroid than nothing at all, if you find they cannot afford a dermatology referral, Apoquel/Cytopoint/Zenrelia, or other topical/antihistamine options are not working well. Remind owners to always give steroids with food, as they can cause gastric ulceration, and warn them of the side effects like PU/PD, polyphagia, potential to cause systemic disease (kidney disease, diabetes, etc.), behavior changes, etc.

- **Oclacitinib (Apoquel) (4-10/10 pruritus scale):** **Apoquel** is a good option for dogs. It is labeled for use at over a year of age. It may help with itch and mild inflammation in cases that have moderate to severe pruritic clinical signs. In patients who are pruritic that are <1 yr of age, Cytopoint is a better option. Steroids can be considered sparingly if they are <1 yr old with severe inflammation and itch. Apoquel works almost as well as prednisone for pruritus and is usually effective within the first 24 hours. The benefit to using it over prednisone is that it does not have the side effects you see with prednisone. It can be started and stopped at any time and used twice daily for up to two weeks in times of a flare-up. If at any point Apoquel is not working as well, then that means there may be a complicating factor present, such as a skin infection. This means their dog needs an appointment to reassess the treatment plan. If needed, you can recommend a trusted client to increase Apoquel to twice daily for a short 7-10 day course in case their dog is having a flare-up. However, ensure they understand that chronic use should be limited to once daily dosing and that they need to come in for a recheck if this short term increase does not improve their dog's clinical signs. Avoid using the newer chewable version in dogs on diet trials.

- Many clients will be resistant to using Apoquel in the beginning, so you will want to have an open conversation with them to choose the best products together for their pet. You can always tell an owner that we can try topicals and antihistamines first, but if their pet remains itchy or worsens over time, then it is time to consider a course of Apoquel or Cytopoint to see if symptoms improve on these medications.
- **Long term Apoquel in older pets:**
  - To date, Apoquel does NOT *cause* cancer. However, if a pet has had cancer previously, develops cancer, or has an existing cancer, it may allow that cancer to grow faster. For any pet that is going on Apoquel long term, we like to inform owners of that. That is important for them to hear because many will want to stop this medication once cancer is diagnosed. Some may prefer to try Cytopoint instead when they hear this, while others will recognize this can occur and still choose Apoquel because it works so well to manage their pet's comfort.
  - Explain to owners that every medication has pros and cons, and Apoquel is a very helpful medication for pets that have moderate to severe pruritus. You need to make sure your owner is aware of its use as a long term medication by knowing what it may do to their pet as they age. The last thing you want is for the owner to get on Dr. Google and read some blogs that scare them, causing them to call back upset as to why you prescribed this medication. Believe us, it happens!
  - Let an owner know that it is very important that their pet get annual physical exams with blood work so that you can monitor their dog's health while on a chronic medication.
  - Apoquel has not been studied at long term usage twice daily. Once daily dosing shows that it is quite safe long term. You may need to remind owners of this who insist on long-term twice daily dosing. The main concern being that twice daily dosing could cause unintentional immunosuppression. Rechecks to rule out secondary infection exacerbating itch is recommended if this occurs. At recheck, you can also recommend switching to other itch relief options if infection is not present along with treating the underlying cause (diet trial +/- referral for environmental allergy testing and immunotherapy).

Examples of two scenarios where we took our patients off chronic Apoquel

- Example #1: Patient with a history of melanoma that was undergoing vaccine treatment. This pet historically responded well to Apoquel. However, once diagnosed with cancer, Cytopoint was chosen instead for atopy flares due to less risk of worsening cancer.
  - **DO NOT use Apoquel in patients with a history of cancer, as there is a possibility it can make it worse due to how it impacts the immune system. Cytopoint, antihistamines, etc. can be safer choices.**

- Example #2: Both of us have had a situation where a skin infection was not clearing up while the dog was on Apoquel. Once we got the patient off Apoquel and transferred over to other anti-itch therapy, we were able to clear up the infection.
  - **Be mindful that occasionally some dogs on chronic Apoquel can develop infections that do not clear up while on it.**

- Lokivetmab(Cytopoint) (3-8/10 on pruritus scale): This **injectable option** works well, and it is great for owners who do not wish to give their dog a daily medication. It controls pruritus only, but does NOT reduce inflammation. It is also good for those that have adverse gastrointestinal side effects from oral medications. It can take a 1-2 days to kick in, . To our knowledge, there are no current age restrictions or medication contraindications with Cytopoint making it a good choice for most itchy dogs. It has even been used with chemotherapeutics.. However, always have your clients follow up with their oncologist to be sure.. Cytopoint controls itch similarly to Apoquel, so they are not typically used together, but it is safe to add on with the other for additional itch relief of challenging cases if the client is aware of additional costs. Some dogs respond better to one or the other due to their slightly different mechanisms of action. If your case has significant inflammation, Cytopoint may not be effective. In cases that are on chronic steroids, Cytopoint is a good option as a steroid-sparing drug.
  - Cytopoint lasts anywhere from 4-8 weeks, and some clients will even feel it works up to 12 weeks. We tell owners to put an alert in their phone at 4 and 8 weeks, so that they can monitor their dog clinically to see if they

notice when pruritus comes back. This allows them to monitor for when their dog may need the injection again. This medication is always better if administered BEFORE the itch comes back, as it may not be as effective if they start scratching leading to inflammation and secondary infections.

- Explain to owners that Cytopoint works well in roughly 80% of patients, but that every now and then it does not work as well in others. Due to this, we still recommend trying it if they have not yet to see how their dog responds to it.
- Rechecks are helpful in evaluating response to therapy and to ensure the skin infection has resolved if one was present initially. It also allows you to touch base to ensure compliance is appropriate and reiterate the 4-8 week time frame Cytopoint covers so that owners ensure they keep up with the injection the moment it is needed again.

Cytopoint tip

Cytopoint can take 1-2 days to work so for really itchy patients, you may want to give something additional for a few days to make your patient comfortable. Options include...

- DexSP injection (0.1 mg/kg IV or SQ): This covers the first 24 hours of itch and decreases inflammation right away.
- Oral medications: Options include prednisone, Temaril P, or Apoquel based on severity. Your patient may only need enough for 48-72 hours.

Dr. Jeff's perspective on this tip: I would recommend reserving this tip for rechecks when the owner notices the Cytopoint takes a few days to work. I think most cases that are trying Cytopoint for the first time don't necessarily need extra meds to bridge the gap, which also reduces time in the exam room/additional explanations. I do think it is correct that Cytopoint sometimes takes a little while to kick in, but I have found that treating secondary infections or topical therapy in general is sufficient enough at reducing itch while it begins to do its job.

- **Ilunocitinib (Zenrelia):** This is the newest itch relief option on the market. It is in the same class as Apoquel, but has a slightly different mechanism of action. Like Apoquel, it is also labeled for use over 1 year of age. It works well for pruritus and also has mild anti-inflammatory effects. Patients who have failed other antipruritic medications or who are "stuck on steroids" have been transitioned to Zenrelia with excellent efficacy. It can be considered as a first line option.
    - **Drawbacks:**
        - Like Apoquel it is not recommended in patients with a history of cancer.
        - It is also currently recommended to be withdrawn 1-3 months prior to and 1 month after routine vaccinations in the United States. Interestingly, many other countries do not have this withdrawal recommendation. We recommend updating yourself on the latest studies and following updates from the manufacturer (Elanco) as label updates are currently in progress and thus far announcements appear positive. The "safest" option is to use this medication in fully vaccinated dogs to assess itch control (such as a 1 month trial). If the client would like to stay on Zenrelia because it is working well for itching, then you will need a withdrawal plan with other antipruritics if you choose to follow the recommended label strictly on a long-term basis.

- **(Cyclosporine) Atopica:** This is an older anti-inflammatory/antipruritic medication that is not used as often for allergies due to the newer options mentioned above. It is typically reserved for more severe instances or refractory cases where your patient is not responding well to the above therapies. We do not use it very often due to its side effects and that it can take up to 30 days to work. It is most commonly used for immunosuppression in your more severe skin cases, such as auto-immune diseases.

4. **Prescription diets:** A strict prescription elimination diet trial for 8-12 weeks is recommended for all pruritic patients as this is the ONLY way to definitively rule out food allergy. This should be followed with a diet rechallenge period for 2 weeks (reintroduction of the old diet). Flare during 14 days of old food being reintroduced confirms food allergy. In addition, going back to the prescription diet 100% should resolve a mild to moderate flare.

a. Based on new research, there are now three categories of diets that can be used for diagnosis (hydrolyzed, novel protein and elemental diets).
    i. It is **always best to rule out a food allergy in pruritic patients prior to referral,** as many dermatologists will need to rule out food allergy prior to environmental allergy testing. Any of the 3 categories can be used to rule out food allergy.
        1. **Hydrolyzed protein diets:**
            a. Work well in most cases. Prioritize these especially in cases where you do not know the past diet history (example: rescue dogs).
            b. Consider: Royal Canin Ultamino, Royal Canin HP, Purina HA (vegetarian formula only), Hill's Z/D
                i. Note: HP has a puppy formulation.
        2. **Novel protein diets:**
            a. These diets can also work well. They should only be used if the owner knows ALL past history of previous foods as you will want to select a protein the patient has never had before. (example: a dog that has always eaten chicken and rice kibble can try a prescription Kangaroo diet). Pro tip: avoid proteins that may cross-react. For example: A patient who has had chicken in the past, should avoid ALL poultry for their novel protein selection. Many dermatologists also avoid venison in patients who have had beef.
            b. Consider: Rayne Nutrition Kangaroo, Alligator and Rabbit.
        3. **Elemental diets:**
            a. This newer category utilizes purified amino acids to avoid the immune response that leads to pruritus from food allergies.
            b. They are unique and separate from hydrolyzed and novel diets.
                i. Instead of utilizing protein molecules like other diets, elemental diets add the building blocks of proteins (amino acids) which are extremely small molecules that avoid food allergy flare in the gut. Fortunately, the body can readily absorb the amino acids and use them like normal.
            c. The only elemental option available on the market currently is Purina EL Elemental. One study showed a prevalence of 40% of dogs with food allergy (greater than 20% seen in past food allergy studies) making it an excellent first line choice for any elimination diet trial.

i. The largest size bag is 16.5 lbs currently, so it may be best suited for smaller and medium size dogs for owners with cost concerns.
ii. This diet also supports puppy growth.

ii. If your patient's pruritus has less than 50% improvement on a diet trial, then they are likely atopic. The elimination diet trial should only be skipped in cases where your patient has exclusive seasonal pruritus (such as pruritus ONLY in the spring/summer). This type of case can also be considered atopic. In atopic cases, consider atopy diets. We love these diets for owners who want to take a more natural approach because they can work very well. Oftentimes, you can manage mild cases with a derm diet alone! These diets are aimed at strengthening the skin/coat barrier through vitamins, minerals, and antioxidants. We use Purina DRM and Hill's Derm Complete a lot. Like elimination diets, these diets may take 2-3 months to show effectiveness.

iii. If your client is opposed to a prescription diet, an over the counter diet we offer is Purina Pro Plan sensitive skin and stomach. This type of diet may help in mild atopic cases. However, it would not be suitable as an elimination diet. It is important to remember that OTC diets cannot definitively rule out food allergy, as many studies have shown that OTC limited ingredients diets may still contain cross contamination of proteins not listed on their labels.

5. **Skin support:** There are **many supplements** hat can help the skin and coat. Most commonly, we use omega 3 fatty acids to help decrease inflammation and improve the skin/coat barrier. Brands we like are Nutramax Welactin or Bayer Pet Protect Free Form Omega 3 Fish Oil because both of these products dose appropriately to their pet's weight. There are now more vets trained and familiar with additional nutraceutical and homeopathic options, if your client wishes to explore this route more.

Treatments for paw pruritus (paw licking)

1. Anti-itch medications.
2. Wiping paws.
3. Additional topical treatments.
4. E-collar.
5. Systemic antibiotics/antifungals when warranted.

- Choose **one of the anti-itch medications** mentioned above such as Apoquel, Zenrelia, prednisone, or Cytopoint based on severity of pruritus +/- severity of erythema/inflammation. Reminder, Cytopoint does not control inflammation. For Apoquel, we start BID for 7-14 days depending on the itch level, and then go to SID until recheck or for maintenance on an as needed basis. In mild pruritus cases where you also want some inflammation relief, Apoquel can also be started SID to avoid the "rebound itch" sometimes noted when reducing from BID to SID or Zenrelia could be tried.
    - Examples:
        - Pruritus scale of 8/10, we will prescribe Apoquel for about 14 days BID, and then go to SID for maintenance.
        - Pruritus scale of 4-6/10, we will prescribe Apoquel for about 7 days at BID, then go to SID, and then as needed.

- **Wipe paws** each time they come in from outside. Medicated wipes are helpful, and many cases benefit from this. Many are formulated with chlorhexidine and an anti-fungal which are preferred if secondary bacterial or yeast infection is present. Our favorites are Ketoseb or Malaseb wipes that the owner uses every 12-24 hours. If the wipes get irritating, the owner should decrease their use to every 1-2 days. Wipes are easy for owners to use and helpful in both bacterial and yeast infections. Longterm, we have owners switch to baby wipes when coming in from outside to wipe off any allergens directly contacting the skin. However, cases with recurrent bacteria/yeast overgrowth (confirmed with cytology) can use medicated wipes for maintenance long-term, if needed.

- **Additional topical treatments** such as paw soaks in chlorhexidine or epsom salts can also be useful. The owner can do this by either filling the bathtub with 1 inch of room temp water and applying chlorhexidine shampoo (or epsom salts) to it. Then, the pet stands there for 5 minutes to soak, followed by a gentle rinse. The owner can then wipe their paws to remove any loosened crusts or debris. If just one paw is affected, this same process can be done in a small bowl.

- **Have the owner use an e-collar** until the medications kick in to break the self-trauma cycle. The licking and chewing is what causes the adverse clinical signs, so this step gives the skin time to heal.

- **Systemic antibiotics/antifungals:** prescribe systemic antibiotics/antifungals if warranted based on cytology.

Treatments for crusty skin

1. Gently remove loosened crusts.
2. Choose appropriate shampoo.

- **You must..de-crust!** What are we referring to? Think of that crusty skin that forms as a result of a bacterial or yeast infection. ***Our dermatologist at school would throw a fit if a pet came back for a recheck still coated in crusts!*** She would make us gently 'de-crust' the skin using gentle soaking with a chlorhexidine based product. The idea is that the bacteria will hide under these crusts, so you need to have a plan in place to remove them while the dog is at home taking medications (at home baths are best). From our experience, the infection will not go away if the crusts persist on the skin. We will often do a gentle 'de-crusting' in the clinic as reasonable. *This should only be aimed at removing loosened crusts.* Nothing should be forced here and we do not rub lesions raw. Send the owner home with a shampoo to continue this process at home once or twice a week as directed.
    - **Dr. Jeff's thoughts on de-crusting:** This is another personal opinion. I usually don't focus on specifically decrusting, but it is case dependent. If there is a case with confirmed secondary infection on cytology, then bathing (like listed in the

next paragraph) is great, and any crusts that are falling off from routine bathing are safe for "decrusting'. However, sometimes crusts are secondary to other conditions like pemphigus and if they're removed you could miss the diagnosis on biopsy.

- **Shampoo, shampoo, shampoo**...Choose an appropriate shampoo. Ingredients are very important. A 2% chlorhexidine based shampoo will work well for routine bacterial infections. A 3-4% chlorhexidine shampoo is efficacious against resistant Staph infections. Most antifungals such as miconazole or ketoconazole included in the shampoo will work for Malassezia. Bathing twice a week is a good place to start. The bottle will give the owner an easy description of what to do, but the goal is to allow the lather to sit for 10 minutes of contact time before thoroughly rinsing. Any lightly adhered crusts that are gently falling off on their own can be removed. Firmly attached, tightly adhered crusts should never be forced off. After bathing, the owner will need to dry the pet well and tell them to be careful not to put collars on too quickly, as this can keep moisture along the skin worsening infection. If the owner is too busy, have them set up these appointments at the groomer, and be sure the instructions are on the shampoo bottle.
    - **Side note:** For those owners who cannot bathe their dog frequently, then you can recommend once weekly bathing with Douxo Pyo chlorhexidine mousse massaged into the areas the rest of the week. They will need to work the mousse into the skin for it to be effective.

STEP 4: Client Communication

We have broken down the communication points you will want to highlight based on the type of appointment you are having below. The truth is that allergies are one of the MOST important conditions for setting up client expectations early in order to get the best success, compliance, and to prevent complaints. Dermatology is one of the most common areas for client complaints due to frustration, and clients will often get second and third opinions if they become frustrated and are not made aware of the lengthy process involved in management of their dog's skin. Documenting and clearly communicating the following points is really important. Most often, it is a lack of communication that causes the complaints. Some owners have unrealistic expectations, which is why communicating clearly here is even more important.

- **First time offender:**

Client communication summary for first time pruritic dog

- "Put out the fire". Focus them on the task of getting rid of infection and controlling itch.
- Discuss that itching leads to infection and is often secondary to allergies or ectoparasites.
- Discuss some dogs have this infrequently, while others will come back and be repeat offenders.
- Set expectations for a recheck regardless of improvement. Ask to call if not improving. And let them know for some pets where this becomes recurrent, dermatology consults are warranted.
- Discuss that an elimination diet trial is the next step if pruritus recurs, especially for puppies!

  - **Focus the client** on the immediate task, which is getting rid of the infection and reducing the itch.

  - **Discuss that you suspect this is secondary to allergies +/- ectoparasites,** and briefly dive into the three most common types of allergies (food, environment, flea).

  - **Dogs with allergies come in two main varieties:** Most fall into "nonseasonal" (itchy all year round) or "seasonal" pruritus (itchy only in warmer months, with no need for meds in winter). Since it is the first time we are seeing their pet for these clinical signs, suggest that we keep our focus initially on clearing the infection and assessing response to therapy. Their dog may respond well and not have another issue for months or even a year.

  - **Set expectations!**
    - **Recheck: Their pet DOES need to come back for a follow up in 10-14 days regardless of if the infection appears resolved or not.** Explain that often they still have bacteria or yeast that you can find microscopically, so that

is why you are seeing their dog back. The recheck visit will also be where you focus your discussion on the possible causes in more detail as well as the preventative measures you want to take for maintenance as most cases of allergy are chronic and recurrent. Being proactive will reduce long-term suffering for the client AND your patient.

- **If the pet is NOT responding to treatment, tell the owner to call sooner** because you may need to discuss further diagnostics in order to adjust or change medications as well as check to ensure compliance is present. However, the majority of pets will improve with this initial plan.
- **Let owners know that when pets have repeat problems or when clinical signs do not respond to traditional therapy, some will benefit from a consultation with a dermatologist.** We do not elaborate much on this at the first visit, but it is just said here to prepare the owner for what may be needed in the future. Continue to guide them that the initial goal is getting control of the current clinical signs since it is their first time having these symptoms.
- **Set the expectation that it is not common to get the itch down to a 0-1/10.** Relate this to human allergies, as many people understand this comparison and how allergies can get worse each year. We manage them, but they are not curable . Tell them that your goal with their pet is to reduce the itch by 50% which clients considered well managed in several studies and some pets get the itch down to a 2-3/10, which is considered "normal dog itch" in many studies. This expectation is Important, and if not communicated, may lead to frustration.
- **First time allergy visit with a puppy:** You should still treat the puppy like a first time offender with treatment, but it is important to have a more serious discussion about a diet change as the next step. Repeat allergy symptoms in a young dog make food allergies more likely, as we know environmental allergies tend to occur due to repeat pollen/dust mite exposure. Environmental allergies can still happen though, and have been reported in dogs as young at 8 weeks of age who did not respond to an appropriate elimination diet trial i. It is never wrong to do a diet trial in a repeat offender puppy, so this is another reminder on the ones formulated for growth: Royal Canin HP (puppy formula) or Purina EL.
- **Pro tip from Dr. Jeff:** If you have time for diet discussion and a motivated client, it is absolutely OK to begin an elimination diet trial on the first pruritus visit for any patient.

- Repeat offender (dog who has a history of pruritus)

Client communication summary for dog with recurrent pruritus

- Focus client on task of getting rid of infection and controlling itch.
- Discuss common causes and suggest starting a diet trial to rule out food allergy.
- Reiterate if no improvement with this, next step is to consider the dermatologist or long-term symptomatic meds.
- Insist on a recheck and set the expectation that multiple rechecks will be warranted.

- ▽ Your focus will still be on getting rid of the infection, but now you are going to give a bigger push for a **STRICT 8 week prescription elimination diet trial** if it has not been performed yet. Your goal with the diet trial is to **rule out an underlying cause for the itch and secondary infection you are treating today**. Make sure the diet trial was performed appropriately if it was done before, which means no outside treats or protein flavored parasite preventatives and that a hydrolyzed/novel protein or elemental prescription diet was used. (Exception: it is OK to give a chewable 3-month Bravecto at the start of a diet trial).

- ▽ **Mention a dermatologist again** to see if there is any interest at this point. We usually prefer to do a referral after an elimination diet trial, as this will help rule out food allergies for the dermatologist. In addition, if the patient is confirmed to have a food allergy and they are comfortable in your care, referral may not be needed!

- ▽ **Insist on a recheck**, so you can revisit the idea of next steps if symptoms are not improving with therapy. It also gives the owner two weeks away to think about if they want to try an elimination diet trial, consider a visit to a dermatologist, or if they prefer to try a longer course of anti-itch medication during their itch season.

- **Any recheck exam:**

    - Always recheck skin cytology, **even if the skin infection appears grossly resolved**. We use this visit to check in, get on the same page with how their dog is doing, and clearly establish the plan moving forward. This appointment is as much about communication as it is about ensuring the infection is gone.

- **First time offender recheck:**

Client communication summary at recheck of first time pruritic dog

- Confirm itch and infection is clear
- Caution owners if this itch returns, to call and come in as you will need to set up a long term plan to look into the underlying cause and start considering next steps such as an elimination diet trial, etc.

    - **Great, the infection has cleared up!** However, we are not out of the woods yet. Discuss allergies again and let them know that if the itch comes back, they will need a **recheck to set up a long term plan.** Consider having them make a tentative 3 month recheck.

    - Tell the client that you are not sure if this will happen again since this is their dog's first time with these symptoms, but often signs will come back at some point. **Have them monitor for seasonality to provide clues** as to the cause and when to treat in the future.

    - It is great to give them **topical medications** at this visit, such as a medicated shampoo, along with an anti-itch protocol for flares. As an example: if you started Apoquel on the first visit, they can restart this at home and call you for recheck at the next flare. In very mild cases, you can send home a dose of an antihistamine, but remember, these only help in 5-10% of allergic pruritus cases.

- **Repeat offender recheck:**

Client communication summary at recheck of dog with recurrent pruritus

- Discuss status of infection and itch.
- Reiterate your long term plan. Bring up diet trial and any interest in the dermatologist Rediscuss possible long term plans you can help them with and discuss scenarios you may encounter (relapse, failure in treatment, long term success, etc.).
- Set up rechecks to assess if infection is still not clearing up (treat 1-2 weeks past resolution of infection).

▽ **Reiterate your long term plan.** Start by ensuring you are treating past resolution of infection. Verify the pruritus scale is at an appropriate level. Then, determine whether you have to switch anti-itch medications, do combination therapy, or add in nutraceuticals to manage them better (building therapies). Check to also make sure topical treatment recommendations were performed and are being utilized, as this is a very important component of treatment.

▽ Often, if we do a course of Apoquel and taper to SID prior to the recheck, the owner will report back that the itch is back. **Quantifying the level of the itch** before Apoquel, during BID therapy, and on SID therapy is important to guide you. An itch of at least 50% improvement is a success to us if the pet seems comfortable and is not causing secondary infection. You can then assess if adjustments are warranted to achieve greater itch relief.

▽ Lastly,has the underlying cause been diagnosed and addressed? Are they willing to do the **strict diet trial or a referral to a dermatologist for environmental allergy testing?** Remember, we always want to do a diet trial first before a referral. Why? This is the first thing a dermatologist will do if you have not done it yet. So, unless the client is getting antsy or being unreasonable, then talk to them about why it is a good idea to do this first with you. It is also important to remember that the sooner you get a dog with atopy in for allergy testing, the better chance they have of responding well to allergen-specific immunotherapy. We love to remind and encourage owners about this in dogs that are chronic offenders.

Final tips on how to make your skin appointments run smoothly

1. Utilize your technician. They can get you a thorough history and start your skin cytology.
2. Confirm history during your conversation with the owner.
3. Perform a full physical exam.
4. Send the owner home with a handout and/or dismissal detailing your treatment plan at each visit.
5. Communicate expectations.
6. Pro tip from Dr. Jeff: Schedule dedicated visits. Allergies are a skin disease/disorder. To provide the best care, encourage itchy pets to schedule a "sick" visit for the skin rather than providing a rushed explanation at the end of a wellness visit.
    - ▽ **What to do in the moment if a client mentions itching at the end of a wellness (or any non-skin) visit?** This would be a reasonable time to offer a 2 week anti-histamine trial and medicated topical therapies. Then, recommend a recheck exclusively for the skin in 2 weeks.

1. Utilize your technician:

    a. **History taking:** Below are seven questions your technician can briefly ask to help you with your allergy history. These answers will get you a basic idea of what is going on so that you can start to formulate your plan.

Seven important history questions your technician should ask:

1. Confirm why the pet is here?
2. Is the dog otherwise healthy? Any abnormal symptoms like C/S/V/D?
3. Current medications and diet?
4. Any recent changes such as diet, recent move, etc.?
5. Is the dog currently on flea prevention, and if so which one, and when was it last applied?
6. Pruritus scale? Get a number 1 out of 10, with 10 the itchiest.
7. Itch or lesions noticed first? Location of itch, when it started, is this new, and have they had these symptoms before?

b. **Have your technician grab a skin cytology for you (tape prep is easiest)** immediately after getting the patient history. This is something you can easily train them to do and discuss with your owner on why it is important. Just like we mention in our otitis chapter, this improves efficiency since you need time to perform the diagnostic. You can also train your technician to evaluate skin cytology and provide results prior to you entering the room.

2. **Confirm history during your conversation with the owner:**

a. Example conversation:

i. *"Good morning! It is so great to see Fido today. So I understand he is here because he has been licking his paws and shaking his ears for the past week? Has this happened before?"*

b. You will be surprised how much it can change from what they tell your technician. Confirm if their pet has had this symptom before and what worked previously. Confirm if there are any changes in food or new treats, as this could be what caused the flare-up.. Lastly, are all pets in the household on flea prevention (including indoor-only cats) and are other pets or humans in the household itchy?

3. **Perform a full physical and dermatologic exam each time:**

    a. Do not forget to look at ears and rears. Have your technician hold up the pet to look at the axilla and inguinal region thoroughly. Look under and around paws and claw beds, even if they are not licking there. On your brachycephalic dogs, do not forget their facial and tail folds. Check the anal glands of dogs biting at their tail or licking around their rectum if warranted.

4. **Send the owner home with a handout and/or discharges detailing your treatment plan at each visit:**

    a. This promotes compliance and lays out the regimen for them in detail in case they did not absorb everything you mentioned that day.

    b. Nearly every visit will also require delving into the three most common allergies: food, environment, and fleas. Early discussion on the types, ways to rule each out, and management strategies will keep the process streamlined.

    c. You can also find handouts that have a brief overview of the three common types of allergies in dogs that you can send home with your clients so that they can understand the process better. Google "veterinary partner" which is powered by VIN. They have some good client facing handouts.

5. **Communicate expectations:** See previous sections for more details. Here is a brief summary.

    a. Allergies are typically a chronic, incurable condition that can be very well managed with a good plan.

    b. Itch goal is 50% reduction, but some dogs get to 2-3/10. We can improve the itch, but full resolution should not be expected. The goal is long-term comfort, not cure.

    c. We must do rechecks and use medications and topicals as directed. Compliance is key!

    d. Always troubleshoot! Discuss that therapies can be effective initially, and then not work as well later in life. Some dogs will also respond better to one therapy over another. Therefore, we may need to add or adjust therapies over time as clinical signs and severity change.

e. Allergic pruritus can be frustrating, so treatment may require an elimination diet trial or dermatology referral in the future if we find their dog is not responding as we would like to our treatment plan.

References:

- Small Animal Dermatology: A Color Atlas and Therapeutic Guide. 3rd Edition. Keith A. Hnilica.
- Muller, George H., et al. Muller & Kirk's Small Animal Dermatology. 7th ed., Elsevier, 2013.
- Fossati LA, Larsen JA, Villaverde C, et al. Determination of mammalian DNA in commercial canine diets with uncommon and limited ingredients. Vet Med Sci. 2019 Feb;5(1):30-38. doi: 10.1002/vms3.125. Epub 2018 Oct 29. PMID: 30375199; PMCID: PMC6376140.
- Tinsley J, Griffin C, Sheinberg G, Griffin J, et al. "An open-label clinical trial to evaluate the efficacy of an elemental diet for the diagnosis of adverse food reactions in dogs." Vet Dermatol. 2023, https://doi.org/https://doi.org/10.1111/vde.13198
- Cox, Allison et al. "Detection of DNA from undeclared animal species in commercial canine and feline raw meat diets using qPCR." The Canadian Veterinary Journal. vol. 61,9 (2020): 977-984.
- Olivry T, Mueller RS. "Critically appraised topic on adverse food reactions of companion animals (9): time to flare of cutaneous signs after a dietary challenge in dogs and cats with food allergies". BMC Vet Res. 2020;16:158.
- Gadeyne C, Little P, King V, et all. "Efficacy of oclacitinib (Apoquel) compared with prednisolone for the control of pruritus and clinical signs associated with allergic dermatitis in client-owned dogs in Australia." Vet Dermatol. 2014
- Miller J, Simpson A, Bloom P, et al. "2023 AAHA Management of Allergic Skin Diseases in Dogs and Cats Guidelines." J Am Anim Hosp Assoc 2023; 59. (DOI 10.5326/JAAHA-MS-7396)
- Forster S, Trout, C. Despa S, et al. "Efficacy and Field Safety of Ilunocitinib for the Control of Allergic Dermatitis in Client-Owned Dogs: A Multicenter, Double-Masked, Randomised, Placebo-Controlled Clinical Trial" Vet Dermatol. 2025, https://doi.org/10.1111/vde.70009

NOTES:

NOTES:

Seizures in Dogs

Reviewed by Dr. Marie Dantio, DVM, DACVIM (Neurology)

It is very important to get comfortable with seizure management because this will be a common disease you manage in general practice. As a new grad vet, you will have appointments with seniors who have well controlled seizures, young epileptics who are not well controlled, and walk-in status epilepticus patients...to name a few. Oftentimes, owners are hysterical in these more emergent presentations, so it is important to keep your calm and get your spiel down so that you can effectively navigate these owners. We will break down everything from differentials to diagnostics to treatment options and more. We want to help you manage these cases with ease in general practice. You will find that many owners are unwilling to seek referral due to financial limitations or advanced age of their pet. Remember to always use your signalment and history to guide you as to what may be the likely cause here.

A summary of common differentials based on age

- **Young dog onset (less then 6 months):**
    - Toxin
    - Infectious (think viruses like distemper, etc.)
    - Metabolic (such as hypoglycemia, portosystemic shunt, etc. rarely nutritional)
    - Inflammatory (GME, etc.)
    - Congenital (hydrocephalus, other malformations like porencephaly etc.)
    - Juvenile epilepsy
    - Idiopathic epilepsy is still on the list- can start as early as 6 months
    - Trauma
    - Etc.

- **Middle age dog onset (1-6):**
    - Idiopathic
    - Toxin
    - Infectious
    - Trauma
    - Metabolic
    - Inflammatory
    - Vascular event
    - Etc.

- **Old dog onset (greater than 6 years):**
    - Intracranial neoplasia (primary or metastatic)
    - Toxin
    - Vascular event- stroke
    - Metabolic (ex: hypoglycemia due to insulinoma, end stage organ failure (think liver, kidney, etc.))
    - Inflammatory
    - Etc.

Dr. Marie Seizure Insight

- Juvenile epilepsy can start in dogs as young as 6 weeks old. Some of these dogs can go into spontaneous and drug induced remission but the overall rate is less than in people with this disease.
- Seizures are often the first sign of a brain tumor in dogs over the age of 7!

Diagnostic plan

- **If neurologically normal**, start with screening blood work: CBC, Chem17, electrolytes, urinalysis, bile acids, +/- T4.
    - This helps you rule out certain metabolic and systemic causes of seizures to get an overall health screen.

Dr. Marie Tip

I do not routinely do urinalysis and bile acids, but it is not wrong to perform. UPC is also something to think of when you have high protein for stroke like events

- **If neurologically abnormal**, then perform the above blood work + further work-up. This can include screening abdominal and thoracic x-rays +/- neurology referral if the owner is interested in determining an exact diagnosis.
    - **Dr. Marie insight:** Consider toxins for some of these dogs, especially if having other systemic signs like vomiting/diarrhea tremors (could try drug testing).

Helpful hints

- Every case that comes in for a seizure should get blood work immediately to help you rule out toxins, metabolic abnormalities, organ injury, etc. as a starting point. You can easily perform a BG on a glucometer if all you can get is a small sample due to the status or size of your patient.
- Memorize or have the diazepam/midazolam dose ready in your phone for easy access if you have a presenting seizure.
- Midazolam is a less expensive alternative to diazepam that can be given intranasally.

Let's break down how to handle a conversation with an owner from start to finish

1. **Confirm that it is a true seizure.**
2. **Discuss differentials for a seizure: intracranial vs. extracranial.**
3. **Set expectations.**
4. **Discuss when medications are warranted.**
5. **Explain when a seizure is an emergency.**
6. **Tell an owner to start a seizure journal.**
7. **Send home with a handout discussing seizures and a summary of your visit.**

1. **Confirm that it sounds like a seizure** with paddling, loss of consciousness, voiding, etc. Many owners will confuse vasovagal or syncope with a seizure.
   - ▽ **Dr. Marie Insight:** Have owners obtain videos or ask for videos. They don't always help but when they are clear cut seizures, it makes it so much easier.

   a. **Recommend that you start with blood work right away** to decrease suspicion of extracranial differentials like liver disease, kidney disease, hypoglycemia, toxins, etc.

   b. **Example:**
      i. *"Mrs. Jones, we have Angel in the treatment area right now being monitored closely. My staff will alert me if there are any concerns while we talk. Can you tell me more about this seizure? What was she doing before the episode? Was she exercising, coughing, or sleeping? How long did it last...what did it look like? Was there any drooling, chomping of the jaw, rigidity of limbs, jerking of limbs, urinating and defecating...how did Angel act before or after?"*
         - ↓ **Dr. Marie tip:** *Ask for the owner's depiction first. Then when done, you can ask more specific questions like those above.*

      ii. *"It does sound like Angel has had her first seizure. I would like to start looking into underlying causes by running some blood work. Are you ok with this? We can have the results back within the hour, while we monitor her closely."*

2. **Briefly discuss the differentials of a seizure, keeping it broad with your two categories of extracranial and intracranial causes.** You can mention what your primary differentials are for their dog. You will then explain next steps and determine if the owner is willing to continue the hunt for the exact cause vs. treat symptoms supportively. This discussion will go something like this...

   a. *"Ok, so now that we have our blood work back, I would like to discuss some causes of Angel's seizures and our next steps. Her blood work helped me to rule out certain causes since it all came back normal. These causes are considered things 'outside of the brain' like low blood sugar, organ failure, etc. At this point, we now need to discuss causes that can occur from 'inside the brain.' Some examples include idiopathic (no known cause), infections, and brain tumors. I know this can sound scary, so I want to guide you to how we determine exactly what is going on."*

   b. *"At this point, we can either continue to dig deeper and figure out the exact cause or come up with a plan to make Angel comfortable. In order to determine exactly what is causing her seizures, I can do screening x-rays here of her chest and abdomen. This allows me to see if any organs are abnormal and look for signs of cancer. From there, a neurology consult will be the next best step because an MRI and CSF tap will allow us to look further into what may be going on inside of her brain. I would have to refer you to a specialist, and they will take great care of you both as we all work together to figure out what is going on with Angel."*

c. *"If you are interested in referral, I am happy to discuss cost as well as the process with you so that you can determine if this is something you want to do. Otherwise, what I can do for you here today is discuss seizures in more detail so that you know exactly what to expect, determine if medications are indicated, and discuss signs you can monitor for in the future."*

Our three big criteria to tentatively diagnose a dog with idiopathic epilepsy:

1. Often have a normal neurologic exam
2. Age of onset typically 6 months to 6 years
3. Blood work is normal, ruling out systemic and metabolic causes

***These suggest idiopathic epilepsy, but there are certain situations when even these dogs have an underlying condition. There are parts of the brain where disease can be present without neurologic signs (silent areas). Idiopathic seizures tend to be rhythmic.

Dr. Marie insight: Determining whether a first seizure onset is idiopathic can be very challenging unless neurologic deficits are present. I have seen dogs with lateralizing neurologic deficits that initially suggest an intracranial cause; however, these findings can also be attributable to post-ictal effects. Use repeat neuro exams and progression to guide you too.

3. **Set expectations.**

   a. Explain how their dog will have seizures again at some point, but it is often difficult to determine at this point what the frequency will be.

i. *"Mrs. Jones, now that we know Angel has seizures. It is important for you to know a few things. Seizures can be unpredictable. Angel may not have another seizure for 6 months, or she could start having multiple seizures next month. Unfortunately, we cannot predict her seizures. Our goal is to work together to decrease the frequency and severity, but it is important to know that unfortunately we cannot eliminate seizures, only manage them."*

b. Many of these dogs can be managed here in general practice, but in some cases it is important to refer their dog to a neurologist if we find that we are unable to manage their seizures well. It is also important to let an owner know that we are happy to send them for referral if they are interested in going, once they have had time to digest this information.

ii. **Note**: If we have a patient that may need a third anticonvulsant drug, we HIGHLY encourage them to consider a neurology consult again because of nuances with seizure management at this point. A specialist opinion on the management plan can be very important at this stage.

4. **Discuss the times when we place dogs on medications and if they are warranted now.** It is important for an owner to understand that not every pet with seizures will go on medications. We will often only place dogs on medications in the following scenarios:

   a. Cluster seizures

   b. Presenting with uncontrollable seizures

   c. Seizure frequency > once a month
      i. Typically 3 in a month is a rough number to tell an owner.

   d. Severe post ictal period
      i. We have both had dogs who walked around acting blind for an hour after seizures.

   e. Or any of the emergent situations mentioned in #5 below

Dr. Marie Tip

I have begun telling owners that it is a balance between seizures and side effects of medications. If their dog has two seizures a month but otherwise a good quality of life, and they don't want to add in medication, then that is fine. We can always add one or another one in the future.

5. **Discuss when a seizure is an emergency.** The following are considered an emergency and require immediate treatment (may mean referral to a 24 hour facility that day):

    a. Three or more seizures in a day

    b. A seizure lasting for longer than 5 minutes

    c. No recovery from seizure behavior before going into another seizure

6. **Recommend the owner start keeping a seizure journal.**

    a. Tell the owner to document the date and time of the seizure. They do not need a video of every seizure, but having videos if seizures change may be helpful. Other helpful details about the seizure include length of seizures, what the movements looked like, and if there are autonomic signs (salivation and urination). The length and severity of the post-ictal phase is also important.

    b. If any of the above scenarios start happening, it could be time to start medications. This journal will be the easiest way for an owner to keep track, as well as be able to see their dog's response to medications once they are started. They will be able to tell if the medications are decreasing seizure frequency or not through qualitative data.

7. **Consider sending home a dismissal with a summary of the above and the following (**to save you time and reiterate what you said because many owners will be overwhelmed)**:**

    a. Print out a handout on epilepsy for the client to read over. There are great ones online if your clinic does not have any. We like to use www.veterinarypartner.com.

b. If sending a pet home with medications, communicate the following:
    i. Expectations when starting the drugs. The goal of the medications are to manage symptoms, as they cannot eliminate seizures.
    ii. Potential side effects to look out for:
        1. Some pets get VERY ataxic and lethargic on the drugs (especially phenobarbital), so they need to expect this to occur. You also need to stress that it could take their pet 2-3 weeks to get used to the medication.
    iii. Follow-up visits are required (short and long term) to assess response to therapy as well as to check drug blood levels along with routine blood work.
    iv. Long-term expectations:
        1. This is an important time to reiterate that seizure medications are needed FOR LIFE. Stress that an owner should never stop a drug without consulting with you first. Warn them that most medications need to be weaned if we opt to stop them later. In rare instances, some patients will go years without another seizure when we start medications, so some owners will not want to give the medication anymore. It is important they know it is not ideal to adjust medications at home.
        2. This is also a good time to mention that some dogs need additional medications if seizure frequency increases again.

How do you explain seizure medications?

Keep it simple. Explain to your owner that there are two categories of medications that we give our patients. Every drug has its own pros and cons. Guide your owner to the choice that you feel is best for their pet based on their health. If you feel indifferent about which drug is best for their pet, then you can give the owner some leeway on deciding, as long as the owner understands the risk of their decision. Some owners will have an opinion and choose based on cost or side effects.

- **Levetiracetam or zonisamide (meds that tend to have less side effects):** These are seizure medications that work about 50% of the time in a patient, but dogs seem to tolerate them better with less side effects. You usually do not need to check levels on these two, but we recommend annual blood work, as with any chronic medication, to keep up with their dog's health. Sometimes, these medications can be cost prohibitive.

- **Phenobarbital or potassium bromide (meds that are often monotherapy):** These medications work well (~80% of the time.), but they can have more side effects. The first few weeks, the dogs are pretty "out of it," so it takes time for their dog to adjust to it. They can also cause organ elevations. Phenobarbital does require checking medication levels and liver values every 6-12 months based on what an owner can afford. These medications are affordable.

Phenobarbital loading dose

Phenobarbital should be loaded if your patient is presenting to you in an emergent situation or with frequent seizures. This is because it can take up to 2 weeks to reach a steady state where it is working well in your patient. There are two ways to load your patient...

- **Oral loading:** This can be performed on those patients who are stable and able to take an oral medication safely. This involves giving your patient a 16 mg/kg dosage orally over 24 hours. For us, we typically will do an ~4 mg/kg dosage every 4-6 hours. At 24 hours, they will start their normal phenobarbital regimen.

- **Intravenous dosing:** This will be performed most commonly in your emergency patients. You are also loading 16 mg/kg but much quicker. There are a few ways to do this...
  - 4 mg/kg IV q2-4 hours based on the level of sedation. Increase frequency to q4-6 hours if your patient is very sedate.
  - 8 mg/kg IV initially if you are struggling to control your patient's seizures, followed by 4 mg/kg IV q2-4 hour until you reach 16 mg/kg.

Dr. Marie tip

I usually only do IV dosing for dogs that cannot take it by mouth. Oral still works pretty quickly.

How do you pick a medication?

- **For older dogs or dogs that have had any of the three emergency seizure situations:**
    - We will often recommend phenobarbital as our first choice because it is highly effective at controlling seizures. You may still give them the option, but if you feel their pet is having moderate to severe symptoms, it is going to be the medication that works best.
        - Dr. Marie insight: My go to is always phenobarbital for generalized seizures. It also comes down to the owner because some owners do not want their dog knocked out. If your patient is older and >50 lbs, they can become knocked out and hard to move with pheno. In that case, levetiracetam might be better. However, if the owner is going to euthanize if their dog has frequent seizures, pheno all the way.
- **For middle aged dogs or those with a history of one seizure periodically:**
    - We often start with Keppra or Zonisamide. They have less adverse side effects that could impact their dog's health long term. These two drugs often control their seizures until they get older, and then we add in phenobarbital as a second anti-convulsant.

A few things to mention to an owner when considering each drug

- **Levetiracetam (20-30 mg/kg PO q8 hr or 30 mg/kg PO BID if XR):** It achieves steady state within 24 hours. High level of evidence based support. Essentially less side effects. Dose escalations may not improve effect, however the drug can be given safely at several multiples above the recommended dose. Little liver metabolism.
    - You do not need to monitor drug levels, though blood work every 6-12 months to assess the health of the patient is important.
    - Dr. Marie tip: As far as side effects go with levetiracetam, I would say that it has less side effects, but it can still have them. I have had a few dogs become aggressive on it, and there are some that have more anxiety. It can also cause other side effects like polydipsia, polyphagia, sedation and ataxia.

- **Zonisamide (5-10 mg/kg PO BID):** This is a sulfa drug, so always ask if anyone in the house has an allergy. Do your due diligence of warning the owner that this drug could cause renal tubular acidosis and very rarely this drug can cause an acute liver reaction (super rare) in their dog. Mention side effects the owner should monitor for such as GI upset, decreased appetite, lethargy, etc. This drug reaches steady state in 7 days. Least evidence in support of its efficacy. There can be drug interaction with phenobarbital since they both use the same hepatic enzymatic system. Therefore, go higher on the dose if used with phenobarbital and recognize it can change phenobarbital levels.
  - You do not need to monitor drug levels, although some neurologists do check a CBC/chemistry 2-3 weeks after starting it. Blood work every 6-12 months to assess the health of the patient is important.
  - The drug interaction with phenobarbital means the dose needs to be increased if the patient is getting both medications.

- **Phenobarbital (2-5 mg/kg PO BID):** Mention common side effects with PU/PD/PP, ataxia, liver enzyme elevation, and that it can become less effective over time (due to levels dropping from liver autoinduction). Warn the owner that their dog will seem disoriented and "out of it" for a few weeks (see below example so you can prevent future phone calls). Rare side effects are dose dependent liver toxicosis and blood dyscrasias (IMHA). Most evidence in support of its use. Dose dependent drug.
  - This drug needs to be loaded the first 24 hours to help the dog reach steady state faster. It can take up to 2 weeks to reach steady state.
    - **Dr. Marie insight:** It can be loaded for emergency settings, but I do not load most patients.
  - Serum levels should be checked after two weeks of its use bc of its serum half life, and it should never exceed 35. It is also important to keep up with blood work along with serum levels every 6-12 months in order to monitor for some of these adverse side effects.
  - **Example:** *"For the next few weeks, Angel will seem really out of it and may not seem like the dog you know...but if you push through that short period with consistency, then your dog will go back to normal as she gets used to the medication. I know this can be difficult, but it is important so that we can prevent life-threatening seizures."*

- **Potassium bromide (35-40 mg/kg PO SID):** Benefits are high levels of efficacy, q24hr dosing, and no liver metabolism (safer in puppies). It has a very long half life enabling you to miss doses without terrible effect. Down sides are PU, PD, but no PP. Sedation and pelvic limb ataxia can occur. Rarer side effects are pancreatitis and skin excoriations. Salt in diet may alter levels.
    - This drug needs to be loaded the first 4-5 days (see Plumb's for the options available) due to the long serum half life. It may take up to 4-5 months to reach steady state.
    - Dr. Marie tip: With KBr, I usually split this into two doses to help with side effects. I start with 10-15 mg/kg every 12 hours. I only load for emergency situations, and I do 100 mg/kg PO a day for 5 days. I also check a level 2 months after starting and then as needed if I think they have toxicosis.
    - You only need to check levels if concerned about toxicity.

***ALWAYS stress these medications are LIFELONG and should not be discontinued suddenly. You can put something on the prescription label because we have both had clients who stop them prematurely when the bottle runs out or if their pet has not had a seizure in a while.

Drugs we avoid with epileptics:

- Isoxazolines (Bravecto, Nexgard, etc.)
    - Dermatologists use Activyl instead

Emergency seizure treatment:

- **Diazepam:** 0.5mg/kg IV. Historically, for quick dosing we have used the rule of "2's" which we learned from our neurologist Dr. Rossmeisl at VMRCVM.
    - ~2 mL for small dog
    - ~4 mL for medium dog
    - ~6 mL for large dog
    - Double these doses if you have to give the dose rectally.

- **Midazolam:** 0.25 mg/kg IV or 0.2-0.4 mg/kg IV or IM (can repeat dose if needed)

- **Off label, you can give Keppra injectable subcutaneously.** This is helpful to know for your patients where you cannot get venous access and are struggling to control a patient with phenobarbital alone. Call your local neurologist or check VIN for dosing.

NOTES:

NOTES:

NOTES:

Thunderstorm Anxiety in Dogs

Anxiety will be a very common conversation you have with clients. There are many causes in dogs, but one of the most common is thunderstorm anxiety. The unpredictability of storms can make things difficult for owners, but fear not as we have many tips for you here! We find it is all about setting expectations with owners and having a multi-modal approach that focuses on a combination of medications, desensitization training, and environmental stimulation. A lot of these tips can translate to other sources of anxiety like loud noise phobias (fireworks, for example), separation anxiety, and sudden household changes (a move, houseguest, new baby, etc.).

Client communication tips to set expectations

1. **Medications do not usually work by themselves.** Be sure to let the owner know medications are best when combined with other calming methods (Adaptil pheromone, Thundershirt, playing calming music, keeping shades down, feeding them with a LickiMat Buddy or Kong, etc.) and desensitization training. You can find many handouts online or discuss this method of training with your client so that they can do their own research. If your patient is not improving with these methods, it is important to mention a professional trainer or veterinary behaviorist may get the best results.

2. **It is always best to have the medications on board well BEFORE a thunderstorm starts.** This is CRUCIAL to explain to your client. They will need to keep up with the weather, and try to give the medication roughly 1-3 hours before it may start. Oftentimes, storms are in the afternoon or early evening, so they can try to give it mid to late afternoon for best results. Explain to them that it is a lot harder to 'calm' a dog down after they are worked up.

3. **Medications work differently in each pet.** Make sure your client understands this about medications, so the expectation is set that if one medication is ineffective, then we may

need to adjust our plan. You can either adjust the dose, try a new medication, or add in a second/third medication. Make sure to tell your owner that they should not adjust the dose on their own, as it may not be appropriate for their pet.

Thunderstorm phobia: 3 quick and easy medication protocols

Option 1:	Option 2:	Option 3:
▶ Adaptil Spray, Thundershirt, calming music etc. ▶ Alprazolam (Xanax) 0.1 mg/kg PO every 6-8 hours **Example:** 50 lb dog: Alprazolam 2 mg tablet: Give 1 tablet every 6-8 hours on day of thunder-storm. Best given before thunderstorms start.	▶ Adaptil spray, Thundershirt, calming music, etc. ▶ Trazodone 8 mg/kg PO every 8-12 hours throughout day of thunderstorm or at least 1-2 hours prior ▶ +/- Alprazolam dose from option 1 if still not enough **Example:** 50 lb dog: Trazodone 100 mg tablet: Give 2 tablets by mouth every 8 -12 hours on day of thunderstorm. Best given before thunderstorms start. **Trazodone has an easy/fast dosage chart in Plumb's too!**	▶ Adaptil spray, Thundershirt, calming music, etc. ▶ Sileo (see dosing chart) applied to the inside of a dog's lip (The owner needs to wear gloves.). This is basically dosed by the 'dot' based on the dog's weight. A video is available online to show owners how to dose the 'dots,' and there is also a handout you can print. **Example:** 50 lb dog: Sileo (0.09 mg/mL): Give a 6 dot dose 30-60 minutes before the thunderstorm. Dose can be repeated in 2-3 hours if needed. Wear gloves.

NOTES:

NOTES:

Urinary Tract Infections in Dogs

Reviewed by Dr. Jessica Romine, DVM, DACVIM

Urinary tract infections are one of our favorite conditions to diagnose and treat. There is a pretty succinct formula to this disease, and once you get down how to communicate your findings to clients along with when to do the appropriate diagnostics, you will like them too. We will start by going over our general approach with you and then will discuss more specific examples.

General approach to UTI's

Step 1: Determine if your case is a simple or complex UTI. This will determine your work-up at this visit.

Step 2: Initial diagnostics–urinalysis (to confirm you have a UTI).

Step 3: Communicate and pursue further diagnostics, treatment, and recheck.

STEP 1: Determine if your case is a simple or complex urinary tract infection

The very first question we ask ourselves when coming across a urinary tract infection: Is it simple or complex? We can start thinking about this even without urinalysis results by using the history and signalment to guide us. This will allow you to start prepping in your head exactly what diagnostics and conversations you will need to have with owners at this appointment.

- **Simple UTI:**
  - Commonly a female dog
  - Age
    - **Tip from Dr. Jess:** If it is a very young puppy (<6 months, before 1st heat), it could be puppy vaginitis, which does not always require antibiotics. Oftentimes, it can self-resolve without messing up their microbiome. You will typically see white to yellow vaginal discharge, and they are not usually urinating frequently or having hematuria. It can occur as early as six weeks old and usually resolves with their first heat cycle. The discharge may be the only symptom, however some pups will lick excessively, causing inflammation or dermatitis of the skin around the vulva. True puppy vaginitis is a benign condition and does not need systemic treatment because with cleaning the area and hormones it can resolve on its own. I recommend not spaying dogs who deal with vaginitis or UTI as puppies until they go through at least one heat cycle to let their vulvas fully develop and reduce chances of ongoing anatomic issues in the future.
  - Has not had an infection within the past few months/year
  - Healthy otherwise

- **Complex UTI:**
  - Can be found in both male and female dogs
    - Almost all UTI's in males are considered complex
  - Intact female dog...remember that pyometras can look similar
  - Female dog going through a heat cycle can mimic an infection
  - Recurring infection that is not resolving with treatment
  - >3+ UTI's within a year
  - Systemically ill (signs of abdominal pain, lethargy, vomiting, straining, difficulty urinating, etc.)

Simple UTI causes:	Complex UTI causes:
▶ Hooded vulva ▶ Recent bout of diarrhea ▶ Being a girl in some cases (anatomy) ▶ Lack of voiding for an excessively long time (such as when boarding)	▶ Hooded vulva (severe enough to keep causing a recurring issue) ▶ Urolithiasis ▶ Bladder or urethral tumors ▶ Resistant infection ▶ Systemic diseases such as kidney disease, diabetes, cushing's, etc. ▶ Prostatic disease ▶ Diskospondylitis ▶ Congenital abnormalities like ectopic ureters, patent urachus, etc. ▶ Urethral incontinence

Step 2: Initial diagnostics–urinalysis

Confirm you have a UTI: The first thing we do is confirm our patient has a UTI with a urine sample. School teaches you to always perform a cystocentesis, and yes...this is important. However, it can be very stressful for some pets. Many times there will be a high number to too numerous to count WBC + bacteria +/- hematuria, so you can often easily diagnose with a free catch sample. A cystocentesis is most important when you have a complicated infection, as you may need to culture the urine to get more information.

- A good rule of thumb is that you should perform a cystocentesis for urinalysis if your patient is tolerant of the procedure or if you have suspicion of a complicated infection. For a complicated infection, place urine in two sterile tubes so that one can be a "hold for culture."

Hurdles that can slow you down at this point:

- Bacteriuria with no pyuria
- UTI with crystalluria
- Crystalluria with no UTI
- Dilute urine (hyposthenuria to isosthenuria)
- Hematuria with no pyuria

- **Bacteriuria with no pyuria:** In asymptomatic dogs with subclinical bacteriuria, the general rule is NOT to treat. There are a few exceptions to this depending on the type of bacteria. This is a good time to consult with an internal medicine specialist at Idexx or Antech to see their opinion on the bacteria present, especially if you performed a culture and sensitivity test. Currently, we find the following approach reasonable:

    - If you find mild to moderate bacteriuria in an asymptomatic dog, consider benign neglect (if mild), while having the owner monitor for urinary signs. Consider a repeat urinalysis in a few months if you are concerned or if the owner wants to be thorough. However, if the dog does have abnormal clinical signs (PU/PD, etc.), symptoms of a UTI, or a history of kidney disease, then a urine culture should be considered as the next step to guide you further.

    - **Example one:** Dr. Tarantino found a moderate amount of rod shaped bacteria on a cystocentesis sample of urine from an asymptomatic older dog on senior blood work. Due to this, she opted to culture the urine, which grew E. Coli. She consulted with the internal medicine doctor at Idexx who recommended treating, and then to retest upon completion of antibiotics. The data and recommendations on this are continuing to evolve right now.

    - **Example two:** Dr. Gray had a patient with hind limb paralysis from I.V.D.D. who gets her bladder expressed regularly. She has her urine checked every 3-6 months due to the owner wanting to be thorough, and the last two samples showed bacteriuria with no pyuria. Dr. Gray opted to culture the urine, and it grew Enterobacter cloacae. It was resistant to all but two antibiotics that needed to be given intravenously. The specialist at Idexx said that most likely the body has recognized this bacteria as "normal" without clinical signs. The recommendation is not to treat since there is no active inflammation. We monitor her for abnormal signs like an odor to the urine to flag the owner to a possible change.

- **UTI with crystalluria:** Sometimes, you will find crystals in the urine sediment with a concurrent urinary tract infection, and your patient will often have appropriate clinical signs (stranguria, pollakiuria, etc.). With simple UTI's, we treat the infection first and then recheck a fresh urine sample upon completion of antibiotics to see if the crystals are still present when the infection has resolved. It is best to run the urine right away in the clinic, since we know crystals can form at room temperature when urine sits out. If crystals are still present and/or the dog remains symptomatic for the crystals (stranguria, licking vulva, etc.), then consider placing your patient on a urinary dissolution diet for management and follow up to see if improvement is noted within 2-4 weeks. If you have evidence of a complex UTI, then we are more inclined to rule out stone formation from the crystals with x-rays first.

    - Here is a refresher on the three most common reasons to see crystals in urine:
        - Due to the UTI itself. Urine pH change can cause them to form.
        - Due to sample handling. The urine sample sat out too long such as in the fridge at the owner's home or in transport to the lab.
        - The dog is a true crystal/stone former. It could be due to an underlying genetic reason or a variety of other reasons based on the crystal or stone type present. See chapter on urolithiasis for more information.

- **Crystalluria with no UTI:** These dogs will either be symptomatic or asymptomatic. For example, you may find crystals in the urine when you run annual blood work and UA on your patient that was sent out to the lab. If there are no clinical signs to fit with these crystals, then we do not get too excited about them. If there are a large amount of crystals, we suggest rechecking a fresh sample in the clinic to be safe. If crystals are persistent or there are clinical signs, consider a work up for a complicated UTI (abdominal x-rays and blood work). Then, consider placing your patient on an appropriate urinary diet based on the results of your diagnostics.

    - **Tip from Dr. Jess:** Remember that you can have crystals without stones and stones without crystals! I pay a lot more attention to struvites and high pH in terms of UTI screening vs. calcium crystals, which are pretty common in acidic or old urine samples and don't mean there is an infection.

- **Dilute urine (hyposthenuria to isosthenuria):** Dilute urine can occur due to early kidney disease, endocrine disease, psychogenic polydipsia, and more. Blood work will help you interpret if there is an obvious cause for this dilution. These dilute samples run the risk of not allowing you to easily visualize your urine sediment, meaning it is difficult to find bacteriuria, pyuria, etc. In these cases, a culture may be indicated with blood work if you are concerned about infection based on clinical signs.

- **Hematuria with no pyuria:** A couple of scenarios may be going on. Remember, there can be some hematuria with cystocentesis and even mild amounts with your free catch urine samples. If this does not explain the hematuria, then it is possible that the urine has a high concentration of red blood cells in it making it difficult to distinguish or find the white blood cells amongst them. Running a dilution on your urine sample can help you visualize the cells better, and we almost always dilute our grossly blood tinged samples from the start in order to avoid this conundrum. Other causes of hematuria include bladder stones, tumors of the urinary system, urethritis, and even a dog in heat can all be reasons to cause inflammation and hematuria.

STEP 3: Communicate and pursue further diagnostics, treatment, and recheck

Simple UTI plan

1. Urinalysis to confirm infection is present.
2. Medical management with appropriate antibiotic choice, NSAID if painful, and treatment of any possible underlying factors like a hooded vulva or perivulvar dermatitis (medicated wipes, grooming, etc).
3. Communicate the importance of a recheck to ensure infection has cleared. Goal is to prevent a complicated UTI.

Simple urinary tract infections most commonly occur in female dogs and typically have the following history: The patient is normal besides the fact that the dog has increased or frequent urination, licking vulva, blood in urine, straining, and/or accidents in the house.

- Diagnostics: Urinalysis to confirm infection. Most common pathogens are Escherichia coli, Staphylococcus spp., Enterococcus spp., Proteus spp, and Klebsiella spp.
    - **Perspective from Dr. Jess:** Most internists I know do not find the in-house Sedivue to be very accurate. Things are often too crowded, and "bacteria suspected" is always read out, etc. If you have time and good training, always look at your own urine sediments, and if not, I think a dipstick in-house is fine. Ideally send your urine sample out for an expert to review +/- culture.
- Treatment:
    - Most common antibiotic choices include **Amoxicillin** 15-20 mg/kg PO TID and **Clavamox** 13.75-20 mg/kg PO BID (or can do a written prescription for generic human Augmentin, which may be more affordable).
    - Consider an anti-inflammatory (such as Rimadyl) as well for pain management, if your patient is straining and licking excessively.
        - Consider an e-collar if licking is causing skin irritation.
    - If the dog has a hooded vulva or vulvar dermatitis, we also start daily to every other day medicated wipes of the vulvar area. Options we like include Mal-a-ket wipes and Douxo chlorhexidine wipes. Make sure to show them to do it. You will be surprised how many owners do not even look back there. We recommend they start doing it for long term management because this is a complicating factor for a UTI that may predispose them to more in the future. We explain that if we find their dog is getting recurrent infections, we will have to rule out other causes of a complicated UTI first but may end up needing to consider an episioplasty procedure.
        - **Dr. Jess tip:** As above, any dog with an early UTI/vaginitis should go through a heat cycle to develop this tissue as much as possible, and weight needs to be monitored to keep more soft tissue depositing in the area

- Grooming can also help in dogs with long hair around their genital regions that can trap moisture.

- **Client communication tips:**
  - Inform the owner of the diagnosis and treatment plan.
  - Go over any underlying causes you may be suspicious of and the plan associated with them. This includes advice about having their pet void more often, cleaning around a hooded vulva, etc.
  - Stress the importance of a recheck visit to ensure the infection is gone. We tell owners that the goal is to prevent their pet from getting a complicated or resistant infection.
    - Let the owner know that if you find their pet has multiple infections within a year, then you may need to dig deeper as to why. You can still be vague here, however, you are preparing them for a complicated UTI if it arises.

Complex UTI plan

1. Urinalysis to confirm infection is present.
2. Choose next diagnostics based on what is appropriate for the dog's clinical signs.
3. Medical management with appropriate antibiotic choice, NSAID if painful, supportive medications like antiemetics if indicated, and treatment of any possible underlying factors like a hooded vulva or perivulvar dermatitis (medicated wipes, grooming, etc). Consider if hospitalization is indicated for your patient.
4. Communicate to the owner that this is no longer a straightforward infection. Multiple diagnostics and rechecks are needed to ensure the UTI resolves and that we determine what is causing it.

The inciting cause will vary greatly with regards to what is making a dog have a complex urinary tract infection. If you believe you have a complex infection, first decide if the pet is stable and healthy vs. is it a male and/or not feeling well (i.e. lethargic, inappetent, febrile, etc.) because this can indicate a systemic disease may be present. This will guide how aggressive you are with diagnostics and treatment today vs. in the near future.

- Diagnostics: In addition to a urinalysis, you will need to determine if urine culture, blood work, +/- x-rays are indicated for this patient. Very sick presentation...all diagnostics are indicated to best guide you in that moment.
  - **How do you pick which diagnostic to do?:** Let's talk about some different scenarios and what testing we would perform for each.
    - If there is a suspicion that the infection never improved from the previous visit, then a urine culture and sensitivity will be most important. It may just be that the bacteria present is resistant or not susceptible to your antibiotic choice, so this will best guide you.
    - X-rays are an important next step in those patients who have complex UTI's but feel clinically well. X-rays can help you to rule out stones, abnormal kidney size/shape, prostatic enlargement, etc.
      - **Tip from Dr. Jess:** If your hospital has a point of care ultrasound, even if it is not good for full abdomen scans, it is great to be comfortable visualizing bladders and getting a cysto at this point. I recommend scanning both on their back and when they are standing, which can help you tell if things are gravity dependent or not. For example, bladder wall thickening can look nasty, but when you stand the dog upright, you see a stone fall right into that cranial ventral area, so it is more fitting with mechanical irritation from the stone.
    - Any sick patient you see with a complex UTI will benefit from all diagnostics in order for you to be thorough and ensure you are not missing anything: blood work, urine culture and sensitivity, and x-rays.

- Treatment: This will be determined by your diagnostic results.
  - Your urine culture and sensitivity will tell you the antibiotics of choice. If the owner does not allow you to perform a culture, consider the medications used for a simple infection or additional options like cefovecin (0.045 mL/lb SQ), enrofloxacin (5-20 mg/kg PO SID depending on susceptibility), etc.

- Dr. Jess's Enrofloxacin dose go-to is 10 mg/kg SID, but if she is doing a short course, then she goes high dose at 20 mg/kg SID x3-5 days.

- Consider other treatments mentioned in the simple UTI plan like NSAIDs, medicated wipes, etc.

- If systemic signs are present, consider other supportive medications like anti-emetics, etc.

- Remember to always use clinical status to guide you, as some of these patients may also require hospitalization with aggressive therapy. Consider IV antibiotics and fluid therapy in those patients that are not eating well, lethargic, have abdominal pain, etc. that have concern for pyelonephritis or other concerning diseases.
  - **Tip from Dr. Jess:** Take UTIs seriously, especially in geriatrics. There is a lot of evidence in human literature about UTIs in older people, especially with dementia. Oftentimes, they are not having specific lower urinary tract signs but can show worsening of neurologic signs. We see this in geriatric animals as well with hind limb weakness, lethargy, anxiousness, etc.
    - Article for more info: https://www.journalofinfection.com/article/S0163-4453(24)00101-4/fulltext

- Refer to the chapter on urolithiasis for more information on managing complex UTI's along with a complete list and use of urinary prescription diets.

- **Client communication:**

  - Inform the owner that their dog has a urinary tract infection, but due to 'x' it is considered a complex infection. You need them to understand that the infection is no longer straightforward and simple.

  - Explain how this classification means you need to start looking into other underlying causes through additional diagnostics beyond just a urinalysis to figure out why the infection is complex.

  - Suggest your diagnostics starting with urine culture, blood work, and/or x-rays, while letting the owner know the respective cost of each to prepare them. Reiterate what you are trying to achieve with each diagnostic: x-rays to rule out uroliths, etc., blood work to look for systemic disease, and urine culture to look for bacterial resistance and guide appropriate antibiotic choice, etc.

- If the owner approves all diagnostics, this will be very helpful to you because many owners are resistant to diagnostics. If they are not ready to do further testing yet, be sure to just caution them that it may be needed in the future.
- Warn the owner that if the infection comes back, it will be even more important to consider further diagnostics +/- a urinary prescription diet. If you have performed all diagnostics to no avail, an internal medicine consult can be helpful.

Urinary Diet Reminder from Dr. Jess

Remember that a urinary diet does NOT reduce the chance of future UTIs. It is there to encourage water intake, reduce crystal formation, and control urine pH. You cannot dissolve struvite stones with a urinary diet without clearing the infection, and the pH goes high (which leads to struvite formation) when bacteria are producing urease and other factors driving the pH high. It is not the pH causing the UTI, but it is the other way around. If an owner is dealing with UTIs and not stones, spending money on a urinary diet may not be as useful as focusing on other factors or referral.

NOTES:

NOTES:

NOTES:

Urolithiasis in Dogs

Reviewed by Dr. Jessica Romine, DVM, DACVIM

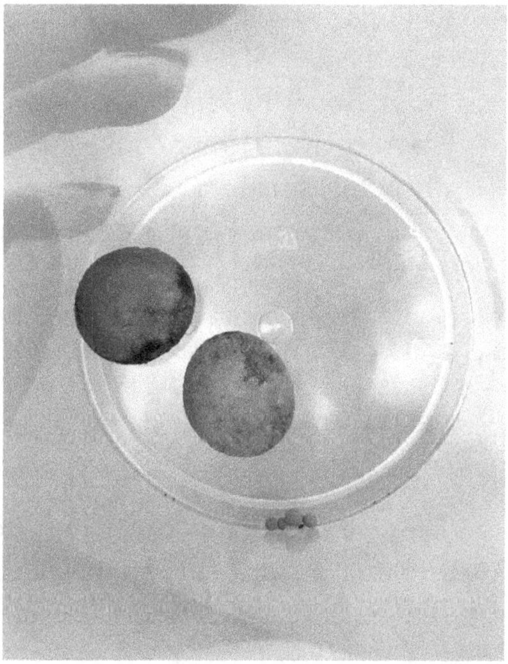

Dogs with bladder stones will present to you in two ways. Your patient will either be symptomatic or asymptomatic. Many times, you will find stones incidentally when you are performing abdominal x-rays or even ultrasound for another reason. Refer to our chapter on urinary tract infections for a detailed discussion on how to work up patients when they are symptomatic to look into underlying causes.

In this chapter, we will refresh you on the types of bladder stones you will see out in practice, the different treatment options available, discussion on use of prescription diets, some tips you do not want to miss with your patients, and pertinent client communication points. Stay up to date by keeping tabs on the Minnesota Urolith Center website. It is a great resource that is updated regularly. Dr. Jess wanted you to know that there is even a free calculator you can use to figure out the odds of a dog having a particular type of stone. We had no idea about this!

Types of stones:

- **Struvite:** These are *radiopaque* and commonly form due to urinary tract infections.
- **Calcium oxalate:** These are *radiopaque* and the mechanism of formation is not well understood.
- **Urate:** These are *radiolucent* and form due to hepatic portovascular anomalies or an inherited alteration of the urate transporter. A few breeds prone to these include Dalmations, English Bulldogs, Black Russian Terriers, and dogs diagnosed with porto-systemic shunts.
- **Cystine:** These are *radiolucent* and form due to an inherited defect in the renal tubular transporters of cystine. A few breeds prone to cystinuria to consider are Newfoundlands, Mastiffs, Staffies, Bulldogs, Labradors, Dachshunds, Basset Hounds, and Irish Terriers.
  - **Dr. Jess note:** This particular stone type is increasing in frequency. It is also well-recognized to be androgen-linked, so these dogs should 100% be castrated when stones are removed. This can often be curative.
- **Compound:** These are a combination of multiple stone types and can be *radiopaque or radiolucent.*
- **And there are more** that are less common you can read about on the Minnesota Urolith Center website.

Our focus will be on the more common stones you will see out in practice. These include struvites, calcium oxalates, and compound stones. As you know, the only way to confirm a stone type is through analysis at the Minnesota Urolith Center.

So, where do you start when you find a stone?

1. Confirm a stone via diagnostics: x-ray, ultrasound, and/or contrast studies.
2. Never forget "the butt shot" on a male dog to assess the entire urethra.
3. Determine the severity of the disease: Is your patient obstructed?
    a. If obstructed, stabilize your patient!
    b. If not obstructed, discuss medical management and dissolution diet options.

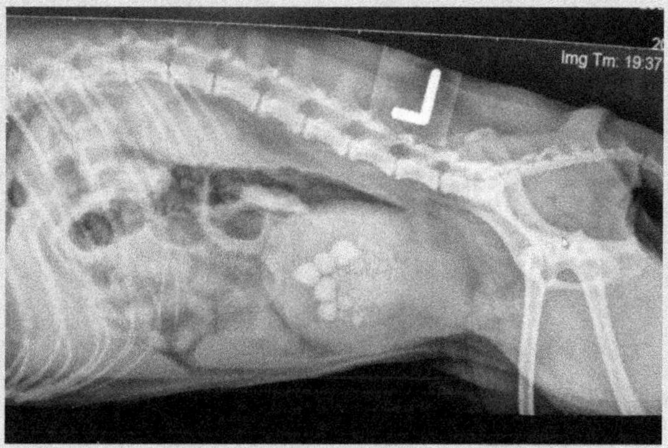

1. Great! **You found a bladder stone.** Radiopaque stones will be visible with an x-ray, while radiolucent stones are found via ultrasound or contrast studies.

2. **Never forget to do a lateral x-ray with the pelvic limbs pulled cranially on a male dog** in order to assess the ENTIRE urethra. Many stones like to hang out near the os penis. You do not want to miss these stones! We call it "the butt shot."

3. **Determine the severity of the disease.** Is your patient symptomatic or asymptomatic? Answer the question of "Can your patient urinate?" If your patient is obstructed, this is an emergency requiring immediate attention. **Here are some tips on obstructed patients...**

    a. Let's start with a cool tip from Dr. Gray:
        i. "I had a female dog that presented to me on an emergency shift with an inability to urinate for 24 hours. She had known bladder stones that were being treated with a dissolution diet. When I palpated her bladder, it was huge and painful. I performed a rectal and was able to feel the stone in the trigone. Without having to place a urinary catheter, I gently moved the stone out of the trigone via her rectal exam. She immediately urinated! This gave time to stabilize her and get ready for surgery."

b. Oftentimes, these obstructed patients need to be stabilized first. Perform lab work to assess for any post-renal health concerns, and then sedate for urinary catheter placement. Many stones can be flushed back into the bladder as you place your catheter, and this ensures you only have to perform a cystotomy instead of a perineal urethrostomy or other more advanced surgeries.

c. Make sure you take an x-ray EVERY time you place a urinary catheter (2 views minimum: lateral and V/D) in order to confirm appropriate placement and ensure all stones made it back into the bladder. Smaller stones like to get stuck around the os penis or are stuck in scar tissue.

d. If you are unable to pass a urinary catheter into the bladder, this patient will most likely require a more advanced surgery like a perineal urethrostomy. This can be a reason to refer if you do not have a veterinarian present who can perform this procedure.

e. While we will not go into detail on a cystotomy surgery here, a good habit to always get into is to pass a urinary catheter during surgery and flush thoroughly in both directions once you have removed all the stones. Dr. Jess recommends that you really palpate all along the os penis and prepuce as well. You can sometimes feel small stones embedded in the tissue. You want to make sure you do not miss any small stones, and this method will help you confirm complete removal while in surgery. It also helps you find pesky stones that may be lodged down in the trigone. Post-op abdominal x-rays will also be performed as a final check before your patient recovers.

f. Gold standard also recommends taking a sample of the bladder wall and sending off for culture. While this is not performed as often as it should, it is an important thing to remember if an owner is open to performing all diagnostics.

g. ALWAYS ALWAYS ALWAYS send the stones off for analysis. This should not be optional because it is the only opportunity you get to determine what the stones are in order to come up with the best prevention plan. Explain to owners that the goal of analysis is to know exactly what the stone is in order to determine the best prevention strategy with diet recommendations, etc. Just because a stone may resemble a struvite (smooth and round) does not mean it is 100% a struvite. The Minnesota Urolith Center will give you a handout with a step-by-step plan to prevent each specific stone, so this is an important point to tell your owner. This is a good time to utilize the calculator from the Minnesota Urolith Center to get started on treatment based on odds while awaiting results because it takes weeks to get results. Don't forget that the Urolith Center interpretation is FREE, and all you have to pay for is shipping.

4. **If your patient is not obstructed,** you have more time to discuss options with your owner. **You are never wrong to try prescription urinary diets for dissolution first.** If the stones dissolve...great! If the stones do not, this conservative plan gives your owner some time to process the next steps.

    a. At the initial visit, show the owner the bladder stones and explain that there are a variety of stone types. Let your owner know that the good news is that their pet is not in an emergent situation but that these stones can be very irritating and cause pain, urinary tract infections, and difficulty urinating. Give the owner all the facts up front because we find that the more time an owner has to process the information, the more inclined they are to follow your plan. They respond best to "*Here is plan A, but plan B may be needed if we do not find Fluffy is responding well.*" An upfront discussion of how surgery may be indicated in the future is important, but the good news to stress is that you have these amazing diets backed by science that may be able to dissolve the stones without a need for surgery. Give the owner a time frame. Let's say 6-8 weeks for dissolution, and then schedule a follow up visit for repeat x-rays to assess progress.

    b. When starting your dissolution diet trial, ALWAYS perform a urinalysis on your patient, along with a urine culture and susceptibility if you find an active infection. You need to address the underlying infection with antibiotics in order to have the best chance of dissolving these stones. Amoxicillin is often a good choice and should be administered the entire period of dissolution. NSAIDs can also be used if your patient is clinical for the stones.

        i. Dr. Jess recommends continuing antibiotics if they are working because bacteria can be exposed as the stone shrinks, causing re-infection if antibiotics are stopped.

c. Never forget to mention to an owner that it can take time to dissolve the stones (anywhere from as long as 4-12 weeks based on the size). In the process, the shrinking stones can put their pet at risk for obstruction. Prep them with symptoms to monitor so that the owner is prepared to act immediately for this complication. Tell owners to actually go outside with their pets and LOOK FOR A STREAM of urine. They should not assume that because a dog squats to urinate, that urine is coming out. Dogs can trick us because squatting does not equal urination and could just be due to inflammation. Dogs have duped owners with this move many times!

d. If the stones are decreasing in size but still present, perform follow up x-rays 6-8 weeks later. If they are unchanged, verify compliance through urinalysis and urine culture and susceptibility, ensure they are taking medications you prescribed appropriately, and that they are ONLY feeding this diet (no cheating with other treats or food!).
    i. **Dr. Jess Tip:** Even if they say they are (or they are), what matters are the numbers. If the urine is not dilute and the pH isn't close to neutral, the stones won't go away. If they were calcium stones with a struvite cortex, you may have dissolved as much as you can.

e. If the stones do not dissolve and the owner wants to address them, you have two options. You can either perform surgery (a cystotomy) or consider non-surgical options. Some specialists and a few veterinary hospitals are performing laser lithotripsy on stones to break them up, followed by endoscopic removal or voiding urohydropulsion. Some dogs are not good candidates for the nonsurgical options due to size of the patient or those with multiple large stones. Make sure to call ahead before sending the pet to ensure they are a good candidate for the procedure.

Quick guide to urinary prescription diets

In this chart, we will touch on the most common diets we use routinely in general practice. As you know, there are many more prescription diets out there, and you can refer to the Minnesota urolith center for the best treatment options for the specific stone you diagnose.

- **Royal Canin:**
  - **Urinary SO:** helps dissolve and prevent struvite stones, reduces risk of calcium oxalate stones
  - **Urinary UC:** helps to prevent urate stones and promotes a healthy immune system and coat health
  - **SO index:** will also be seen on other prescription diets that have this index for dogs prone to forming crystals. Check these diets out if your pet has two diseases you are managing.

- **Hill's:**
  - C/D: helps dissolve and prevent struvite stones, reduces risk of calcium oxalate stones
  - C/D + Metabolic: helps manage weight and the risk of struvite and oxalate stones
  - S/D: strongest diet for fastest struvite dissolution (touts dissolution in as little at 6 days and average of 13 days). Short term diet.
  - U/D: reduces the risk of non-struvite stone formation while supporting kidney and immune function
  - S+OXSHIELD: will also be seen on other prescription diets that have this index for dogs prone to forming crystals. Check these diets out if your pet has two diseases you are managing.

- **Purina**:
  - **UR Urinary Ox/St:** helps dissolve and prevent struvite stones, reduces risk of calcium oxalate stones

An important thing to note is that one diet is only intended for short term feeding. **Hill's S/D can only be fed for up to six months.

For pets with comorbidities: A LOT of other prescription diets now have SO index/S+Ox field claims including some kidney ones, etc. so reach out to your reps to find out which ones are available now. During actual dissolution, you probably want a urinary diet. However, for a controlled dog with other health concerns, you might not need this special urinary diet as much as another diet (say kidney) long-term.

Royal Canin and Hill's also have urinary prescription dog treats, so make sure your owner understands they cannot give anything additional, or it will interfere with the whole point of the dissolution diet trial. These treats, prescription diet kibble, or the canned options can be ways for the owner to spoil their pet.

Final points:

- Once the stones are dissolved or removed, find the appropriate maintenance urinary prescription diet for lifelong feeding if needed. Remember that your struvite stones won't need a urinary diet long term, just control of urinary tract infections.
    - **Tip from Dr. Jess:** A lot of internists only give two strikes with calcium oxalate stones. Repeat offenders go onto potassium citrate +/- hydrochlorothiazide.

- Dr. Jess recommends really focusing the client communication on prevention around the importance of hydration, dilute urine, and urine pH. Discuss how the diet will help this, if appropriate, and discuss a good follow-up monitoring plan. You want to ensure the owner understands how all of this will help to prevent stone formation in the future and their understanding will aid in compliance.

- The ideal diagnostic follow up plan is a urinalysis every 6-12 months with routine blood work, and you can perform screening abdominal x-rays every few years if an owner wishes to be thorough to assess for recurrence.

- Uncommonly, you will find an owner cannot afford surgery or the pet has serious health and quality of life concerns preventing it. In these specific cases where the stones do not dissolve, attempt to manage these patients symptomatically for their stones. Some dogs will never have clinical signs from the stones. If they do, look for infection, treat for said infection, and manage pain with NSAIDs. They should still maintain their pet on a urinary prescription diet to reduce risk of further stone formation.

NOTES:

NOTES:

NOTES:

ACTH Stimulation Test

Reviewed by Dr. Jessica Romine, DVM, DACVIM

Reminder from Dr. Jess

ACTH stimulations are more SPECIFIC (so a positive test more reliably confirms Cushing's), but more than 30% of dogs with Cushing's can have false negatives.

LDDST are more SENSITIVE (so normal makes Cushing's a lot less likely), but you can get lots of false positives due to stress or other illness. Endocrinology is not straightforward!

The ACTH stim test is commonly used for Addison's and Cushing's disease testing. However, more often with Cushing's disease, we are performing both the LDDST and ACTH stim test (can do both tests the same day!). A benefit to the ACTH stim test is that it only takes a few hours to run, as compared to the LDDST, which takes all day. With any test, give yourself a little extra time because you cannot predict a day. Tell your client to drop off for the morning and that someone will call them when their pet is ready for pick up.

- Pick one of the methods below for dosing with your ACTH stim test. EITHER works fine.
- How to perform ACTH stim test:
    - Collect baseline serum sample (pre-cortisol). Be sure to label 'pre' on the blood tube.
    - Administer Cortrosyn (whichever dosing method you pick below).
        - Dr. Jess will often try to use a butterfly catheter for this draw. Pull your pre-sample, and then give the ACTH off the needle into the butterfly without having to do another stick (if the patient cooperates!).

    - Set timer. Collect 'post' serum sample 1 hour later. Be sure to label this sample 'post' on the blood tube.

- ACTH stim timing for dogs on Trilostane: The test should be performed 2-6 hours after trilostane is administered to the dog with a small meal. Aim to be consistent with the time you start the test in future ACTH stimulation tests (i.e. if you start the test 4 hours post pill, then do that next time too).
    - **Dr. Jess Tip:** If you get an unexpectedly low result on a monitoring ACTH stim in a dog who is not acting like they have iatrogenic hypoadrenocorticism at all, the recommendation is to retest 2-4 hours later (so run the test at 4-6 hours instead of 2-4) and often the results are more normal. Because of this, I usually try to not run them before 4 hours post-pill!

ACTH Stim Dosing (pick either method)

Method 1: **Whole bottle method IM**	Method 2: **Calculated dose**
Administer the entire vial (1 mL) of Cortrosyn to the dog (no matter the size). Given intramuscularly. Pros: super simple, gets the job done Cons: If you charge cortrosyn by the amount, then it may be more $$ for smaller dogs.	**0.005 mg/kg (0.25 mg/mL vial) IV** This usually comes out to about 0.2 mL per 20 lbs of dog. Given intravenously. Example: 20 lb dog dose will be about 0.2 mL intravenously (Make sure your cortrosyn 100 mg/mL). Pros: Cortrosyn can be saved in the freezer and thawed before injecting. If you do not use the entire vial, you can save the remaining amount in the freezer, helping with cost. ▶ Dr. Jess says that they freeze it in 0.1 mL aliquots in plastic syringes. They charge for 0.1 mL amounts at a time. They last a long time in the freezer and are stable in plastic, but you can only thaw once. Cons: time to calculate

NOTES:

NOTES:

Interpreting ALKP

Reviewed by Dr. Jessica Romine, DVM, DACVIM

We know Cushing's disease is a BIG topic, so we wanted to include a few more helpful pointers for you at the end of the book. When we first started practicing medicine, we both had trouble knowing when to recommend Cushing's disease testing in dogs. This bonus chapter will provide you with tips on our client communication for an elevation of ALKP as well as the parameters that cause us to start chasing this disease. These two areas were difficult for us as new graduates, and these conversations were often boggled in the beginning.

As you know, there are a variety of causes for ALKP to increase, so the ones we mention below are not immediately life threatening. They are some potential causes to consider when you have your discussion with an owner.

Causes of ALKP elevation on blood work

- It may not be Cushing's disease at this time, though some dogs can develop it later in life (more on this later)
- Gallbladder sludge may be present
- Liver inflammation of open etiology, but no significant disease is apparent
- Certain medications cause it to increase (Do not forget about your phenobarbital, prednisone, etc.)
- Age related remodeling
- Etc.

Interpreting elevated ALKP in patients

So, when is it NOT indicated to look into Cushing's disease in general practice? You will commonly find a mild to moderate elevation of ALKP in your middle aged to senior patients. These patients will often be outwardly healthy with no significant clinical signs, so it can be difficult for an owner to justify spending $600+ on a work-up at this point. So, what do you do? First, interpret ALKP in light of ALT to determine if it may be due to primary liver disease or something else. Next, you can give the option of follow up blood work 4-6 weeks later to assess for a trend. This can be very helpful in guiding you in the short term, especially for concerned owners.

More great resources to help you from Dr. Jess

1. Summary on elevated liver enzymes by Dr. Twedt (in DVM 360): https://www.dvm360storage.com/cvc/proceedings/kc/Gastronintestinal%20Medicine/Twedt/Twedt,%20David_Abnormal_liver_enzymes_STYLED.pdf

2. Common liver diseases (including vacuolar hepatopathy) by Dr. Twedt: https://www.cabidigitallibrary.org/doi/pdf/10.5555/20163255187

What is our cut off value? Well, there is no apparent 'cut-off' value for ALKP that we can find in the literature. Though, there are two scenarios where we feel it is important to discuss diagnostics to dig deeper and get more answers.

1. If you see that ALKP has rapidly increased from previous blood work.
2. If your patient has abnormal clinical signs with an elevation. You may hear your client mention vague clinical signs like morning inappetance (slow to eat in am but eats fine in afternoon), a patient with subtle weight loss, etc.

You will find many middle aged to senior dogs have an ALKP between 200-400 with no outward clinical signs. For us, values under 600-700 without clinical signs, and with only mild increases from year to year, do not get us overly excited. How do you communicate this to an owner? Many owners will get concerned with any elevation on blood work, so we have some tips for you below on how to make this conversation run smoothly. It was a difficult spiel for us to learn and took some time to get comfortable with it in our client discussion. We are excited to give you this new grad "one-up" to make this conversation easy for you from the get go.

Additional things to consider with an elevation of ALKP

Tip one: Verify no recent treatment with steroids (oral or topical) causing ALKP to increase. Verify the owner does not use steroid creams at home that they could be touching to the dog when they pet them. These can absorb and have been found to cause an elevation.

Tip two: If an owner is unsure if their dog is PU/PD, you can always have them measure water intake over a 24 hour period. We ask them to do it for 2-3 days.

Tip three from Dr. Jess: Chronic stress from other things will raise it as well. Things to think about include another chronic illness, high anxiety, dental disease and even severe arthritis. These are cortisol-inducing when constant and incompletely managed.

Client communication for an elevated ALKP in an asymptomatic healthy patient

This is the one value that most doctors hate bringing up to owners because ALKP is a very 'noisy' value that can be elevated due to a multitude of reasons. Your first steps are to always verify the pet has not been on medications recently that could increase it as well as ask about clinical signs that could make Cushing's disease seem likely.

If all clinical signs and outside factors are absent, use this spiel to explain that today's elevation is our baseline and that blood work every 6-12 months moving forward will help us interpret it better. **Here is how we explain it...**

> *"Overall, Annie's blood work looks good. There was one value called the ALKP, which was mildly elevated today at 390. To put it in perspective, I have seen it as high as 2,500+ in a patient. This is a bit of an 'odd value' in that it can elevate due*

many different causes such as liver disease (though Annie's other liver values are normal), gallbladder disease, a disease called Cushing's, old age, and more."

"Since the rest of Annie's organ values came back great, and she is clinically doing well, it is fair to keep tabs on her blood work more routinely. I am not overly concerned about it at this time, but by checking blood work every 6-12 months moving forward, we will be able to ensure it is not elevating rapidly. If in 6 months we see that Annie's ALKP is still climbing, this will give us more reason to look into the cause further with other tests."

Side note: If an owner asks what next steps are, then you can clarify that you typically start with an abdominal ultrasound +/- blood test like a low dose dexamethasone suppression test or ACTH stimulation test. **Here is how we add this in...**

"If you do want to be thorough and look into possible causes now, we can start with an abdominal ultrasound. This costs $250 and will allow us to assess all of her organs in more detail. We may find nothing, but this is a way to dig deeper. If everything is normal, blood work will help flag us in the future to see if things may be changing over time."

Other Testing Tips on Elevated ALKP from Dr. Jess

Tip 1: Totally normal dog? Consider doing a urine cortisol:creatinine ratio as a cheaper next step (vs. ultrasound/ACTH stim) that is an easy screening test before going to more expensive tests. See Cushing's chapter for more details.

Tip 2: Consider testing triglycerides for older dogs with rising ALKP without obvious other clinical signs to rule this out as a contributing factor (that is treatable!) and to try to reduce chances of mucoceles and pancreatitis too. Theoretically, you want a fasted triglyceride sample although more endocrinologists/gastroenterologists are starting to argue that we actually want to see what triglycerides are doing in the normal state - our dogs aren't fasted day-to-day, so we want to know if they are spending a lot of their day with high triglycerides. That being said, all dogs will have a post-prandial upswing in triglycerides that you don't want to accidentally overinterpret. Lipemia should clear within 4-6 hours after eating (peak is 2-3 hours post-meal in most dogs) so I usually say at least 4-6 hours without food.

Eclinpath: Lipemia should clear within 4-6 hours after eating (12 hour fast recommended).

- eClinpath. *Triglycerides*. eClinpath.com. Accessed January 26, 2026. https://eclinpath.com/chemistry/energy-metabolism/triglycerides/

NOTES:

NOTES:

NOTES:

Repeat Calcium Oxalate Formers and the 'GDSE' Method

Practical advice from our local internist: Dr. Jordan Jaeger DACVIM

Reviewed by Dr. Jessica Romine, DVM, DACVIM

One of the problems practitioners run into with calcium oxalate formers is reformation of stones → recurrence of clinical signs and subsequent cystotomies. Unlike with struvites, we know that diet is not entirely reliable in preventing CaOx stones from reforming. This means you find yourself doing multiple surgeries on these dogs throughout their lives and that can be frustrating for the owner, suboptimal for the pet, and even the vet!

Tip for at home monitoring from Dr. Jess:

Consider having owners monitor pH with urine dipsticks at home. They can even purchase a cheap refractometer (around $30-$50 online) so they can check it periodically on their own. Many owners may be more motivated to do this rather than bring samples in constantly.

Some specialists and general practitioners do not recommend a cystotomy if the dog is asymptomatic. Therefore, if you have an incidental finding of bladder stones in a dog that is asymptomatic, it may be best to start by monitoring the dog. If the stones cause a problem in the future, then it is time to discuss options for removal. You may hear varying opinions on this from veterinarians, so it is always best to recommend what you feel is right for the patient and your owner's specific situation.

Dr. Jordan Jaeger, DACVIM, who is our local urinary expert explained a trick to us that he uses to help prevent this conundrum.

Post cystotomy on CaOx or compound stone formers, begin the usual recommendations:

1. Strict urinary diet for life (wet if possible or a gruel)
2. Encourage water intake as much as possible
3. Periodically check urine samples on your patient (at least every 6 months to a year)
4. In addition, he recommends the owner perform the method we describe below once a day for life to help dogs urinate out sediment that is forming. We call it the 'gravity dependent sediment expulsion method.'

The gravity dependent sediment expulsion method

The method goes as follows. Once your patient has healed from their cystotomy, instruct owners to hold their pet upright for 45 seconds before placing them down to urinate. They accomplish this by holding their dog so that they are 'standing up like a person' for 45 seconds in a way that allows any sediment to fall to the neck of the bladder. When the pet immediately urinates afterwards, the hope is that they urinate out small bits of sediment repeatedly over time preventing recollection and stone formation. Daily practice and consistency is essential to success with this method.

This method blew our minds because it was simple and practical! Dr. Jaeger has had really great success with it but stresses a few things:

- Obviously we are NOT doing this in dogs with formed known stones.
- Warn owners it may not work, but we have had really good success with it to date. There are no studies on it yet, so it is a pretty new method.
- The owner needs to do it DAILY and FOR LIFE. Holding upwards for 45 seconds is important to give the sediment time to drop (like a snow globe).
- Warn owners there is a chance (small if done correctly) of obstruction, so ALWAYS make sure their dog is producing a good urine stream. We encourage owners to bend

down and look at the stream and to not just assume the dog is urinating due to their posture (especially important for short dogs).

- The owner should never stop doing this method for a period of time and then just start it up again. This is due to the fact that a stone could have formed in that time frame (can be as short as a few days) and suddenly performing again can encourage blockage.
- Continue prescription urinary diets because that is THE one thing we know can reduce the chance of reformation.
- Also, continue with all other recommendations mentioned above.

NOTES:

NOTES:

NOTES:

When to Refer?

Veterinary specialists provide an amazing service for the veterinary community. Not only do they bring more extensive medical services to our patients to ensure the best care, but specialists are also a great support system for general practitioners. It is near impossible for any one doctor to know it all or to be good at everything. Specialists help you fill in the knowledge gaps when cases become more complicated and will help you manage your patients both in the short and long term. When you start your first job, familiarize yourself with the neighboring specialty and emergency hospitals so that you can see what specialists they have on staff and the services they provide to the community. You always want to offer a spectrum of care to your patients, and many clients will want to seek specialty care for their pets.

So, when should you offer a referral?

Here is the thing. You will get bored quickly if you refer every complicated patient you see. There is an art to "when to refer" because your job becomes less stimulating if you are not challenging yourself throughout your career. As a new graduate, we strongly recommend working up your patients thoroughly prior to referral. Take the step-by-step diagnostic approach to every case similar to what we have outlined in this book for our top twenty cases. If there is a procedure or diagnostic you have never performed before, see if a colleague can help you with it so that you can learn how to perform it under their direct supervision (such as a low dose dexamethasone suppression test, bone marrow aspirate, joint tap, etc.). When you hit a dead end or need advanced imaging, you know it is time to offer referral.

Many clients will not be able to afford referral, so your job as a general practitioner is to offer a broad spectrum of care. If you have a dying, sick patient in front of you, see what they can afford and start your stabilization and diagnostic plan. If you find that this pet is very ill and would benefit from referral, you should always give them the option to see a specialist. We will typically tell the owner that at this point, we can either try to see how their patient will respond with us based on what we know or send to a specialist for further work-up. This becomes a C.Y.A. situation because you want to be able to document you offered referral when you know a patient is very ill. You will have some clients who want to go right away, while others want to wait and see how their pet responds with you first.

How to refer?

1. Work up your patient thoroughly prior to referral.
2. Discuss the cost of referral with your client.
3. Fill out required paperwork and send all records for a complete patient transfer.
4. Review the referral record when it comes back and talk with the specialist if indicated.
5. Follow up with your client to see how their pet is doing.

There is an art to referral. You want to be thorough prior to sending your patient, and there are a few steps you can do to make it a smooth process for all involved.

1. **ALWAYS work up your patients thoroughly.** With any sick patient, you should always be doing blood-work and x-rays (abdominal and thoracic) at a minimum. Do not forget the vet school principle of three views for each study because you can miss something if you do not do this. No "cat-o-grams" either, please! Other testing is added in based on what you are finding or how long you have been working up the patient prior to referral. This step ensures you have a good baseline on your patient because you can look for indicators, such as metastatic cancer, that may indicate a poor prognosis. By screening your patients first, you can have a candid conversation with the owner to see how "all in" they are with referral.

2. Call the specialty hospital and get an estimate for the owner. You can also round them on your case during this call, so they are prepared for the patient if you know they are going to be transferred to them that day. This allows their emergency team to be prepared for the pet's arrival. **Always always always tell the owner what it will cost.** If they are financially limited, you will want to work with the owner to figure out the best plan at your hospital. There is nothing that irks a specialty hospital or owner more than when you send a patient for referral, and they cannot even afford the exam fee.

3. **Fill out the required paperwork on the website for referral and ensure a thorough medical record.** You want to put all medications, dosage, frequency, etc. on the record so they know what the patient is taking as well as good history, all diagnostic results, and your conversation with the owner. You can email all diagnostic results or send along with the owner. Document that you went over the cost of referral and what your next diagnostic steps are for the patient. They may change the plan but that way they can see your thought process.

4. **Review the referral record when it is back.** This is a great learning opportunity to compare physical exam findings, their diagnostic work-up, diagnoses, and treatment plans. It will show you if you had the right train of thought on a case and how they are managing it after diagnosis with follow-ups.

5. **Always call the owner after a referral visit to check in.** This is a great habit to get into because it bonds your client to you by showing you care. This step allows you to get back on the same page with the client on their expectations, and you can schedule the next recheck because many times you can perform the follow-up diagnostics for the specialist. Make sure to always send any follow-up diagnostic records back to the specialist in case they see your patient again in the future.

There are other great ways to utilize specialty medicine as a general practitioner. Many offer virtual consults through companies like Critical Consults. You can call them and discuss your case with a boarded criticalist. There are also specialists at Idexx and Antech you can utilize to go over your diagnostic results if you are stumped on a case. The veterinary colleges and local specialists are also open to discussing cases too, especially if you send patients to them. They will help you with interpretation of results and treatment options. Their goal is to help you if you refer the case, so they will be willing to help you throughout the process.

Just remember, we are a vital part of the referral process. You want to send patients to specialists who have been worked up as thoroughly as possible and ensure that the owner is committed to this next step financially. This teamwork is what ensures our patients receive the best care!

NOTES:

NOTES:

NOTES:

5 Tips to Manage Senior Pets Like a Pro

By Monica Tarantino, DVM
Cofounder of Senior Dog Veterinary Society

When I first started seeing senior pets on my schedule, I used to get nervous. I would look at the chart and think, Oh-no... "*What if they have multiple things going on or some of their diseases are out of check? What do I focus on? What if something's wrong and I miss it?*"

Senior appointments can feel daunting, especially when a pet has ten different issues and an owner who wants answers to all of them in one visit. It's easy to feel like you are falling behind before you even step into the room.

Over time, I realized that senior medicine is not about knowing everything. It is about having a system. Once you develop a structure and rhythm, these appointments go from stressful to deeply rewarding. Here are five things that changed the way I manage senior dogs in practice.

1. Use the Senior Dog Wellness Screening Checklist

2. Have a go-to quality of life scale

3. Take a deep breath and have a plan

4. Categorize your seniors

5. Be a chronic pain champion

1. Use the Senior Dog Wellness Screening Checklist

One of the most common mistakes we can make is assuming that slowing down is normal for older dogs. You will hear it all the time:

"They're walking slower because they're old."
"They sleep more because they're old."

When I talk to owners, I often say, "Yes, aging can play a role in slowing down, but disease and things like chronic pain are common culprits as well." One thing we never want to do with seniors is assume that slowing down is due to age alone because when we do that we can miss the opportunity to help them and that is the last thing any of us want.

Because seniors are prone to so many different conditions or quality of life factors that we can easily miss in a rushed appointment, I created the **Senior Dog Wellness Screening Checklist.** It's the one-page tool I use for every senior wellness appointment. You can download it free at www.seniordogvets.com.

The checklist helps you screen for these things mentioned below. Trust me when I say that no matter how good your history taking skills are, you can still miss these easily in a senior dog appointment. It can be easy to get derailed, especially when you are catching up with regular clients/patients.

- Pain from arthritis or dental disease
- Mobility and function changes
- Cognitive decline (CCDS)
- Incontinence or accidents
- Frailty and stamina loss
- Quality of life concerns

Why use the Senior Dog Wellness Screening Checklist?

I rely on it for several reasons. First, I realized that if I offered all of the validated screening checklists right off the bat to every senior pet parent, they would be filling out ten to twenty pages of forms during a single visit. That kind of volume only adds to overwhelm and takes away from my ability to communicate about the most important topics for their senior pet at this stage.

Instead, I start with the Senior Dog Wellness Screening Checklist to get a quick overview of how the dog and caregiver are doing. From there, I move on to a validated form based on what comes back. This single page gets the conversation started and helps you see right away what areas need the most attention. Once you have reviewed it, you can decide which validated tool to use next, like the DISHAA scale for cognitive decline or the Canine Brief Pain Inventory (CBPI) for chronic pain. The goal is to make screening simple and effective so you can focus on what matters most for that pet and their person.

New Vet Tip: Give your clients the screening checklist before the visit and try to make it something your clinic does for every senior appointment (more on how you can help uplevel your senior/geriatric medicine below). You will walk into the room already knowing what matters most to them and what needs your attention first.

2. Have a go-to quality of life scale

You will have tough appointments with seniors where quality of life comes up. Every senior dog owner eventually asks, "How will I know when it's time?"

Have a go to quality-of-life scale ready. My favorite is the **Lap of Love Quality of Life Scale** (https://www.lapoflove.com/how-will-i-know-it-is-time/lap-of-love-quality-of-life-scale.pdf) because it is simple and it gets owners thinking about both the pet's comfort and their own emotional strain.

Sending this home or reviewing it together during an appointment helps clients track subtle changes and opens the door to honest conversations. It gives you and the client shared language when you talk about decline, good days, or what comfort looks like for their pet.

New Vet Tip: Don't wait until the final days to introduce this. Start talking about end of life planning early with clients even before they're ready and being gentle but candid about it. I usually say, *'It's the thing we don't want to think about but is also so important for us to start thinking about because just like we want to create a good life for them, we also want to create a good death which means starting to talk about it.'* Bringing it up early builds trust and makes those end-of-life discussions much less overwhelming later. If you think your owners may like a course on it, I also have a mini-course for pet parents you can refer them to called, 'Is it Time?.'

3. Take a deep breath and have a plan

Some senior visits can get messy. The owner has a list of fifteen problems, and you have appointments scheduled every 15-30 minutes. Another scenario? They show up for what is supposed to be a wellness exam and the dog has lost thirty percent of its weight or is suddenly in respiratory distress. (All things that have happened to me.)

In those moments, take a deep breath. I suggest always starting every exam (but especially senior pet exams) by simply observing the dog from a distance and then hone in on what matters most that day. Make sure breathing looks normal or if it doesn't (as in some of my more chronic pulmonary hypertension dogs, etc.), check in with the owner on what they are seeing at home and if breathing looks normal to them. Remember, even with stable senior dogs, you can't fix everything at once, and that is okay.

When I am in that situation, I focus on two things first:

- What's most important to the **patient's** well-being and comfort right now (even if it's not on the client's radar)
- What's most important to the **client**

I encourage clinics to book **30-60 minute senior wellness visits** based on the patient's needs, but I know many practices are not there yet. If you are working within tighter time limits and a pet comes in with multiple concerns, narrow the focus. Choose the **top 2-3 priorities** for that visit. I say them out loud so the owner knows I have heard every concern and that we will get to the rest in follow-up visits. Trying to cover everything at once creates confusion and overwhelm. Narrow the focus, document what you're deferring, and make a recheck plan. Here's an example of what I say:

> *"Today, let's focus on his diarrhea, slowing down and appetite changes. Then we'll schedule a follow-up to go over the bumps you found and cognitive changes you are noticing."*

New Vet Tip: Setting limits helps you properly check out each concern and that is usually how I pitch it to owners. I want to make sure we give the needed time for each of these and so today, I think it is best we focus on a, b and c and work on those. Then, I want to recheck and talk more thoroughly with you about x, y and z. Clients respect it when you show them you are being intentional, not rushed.

4. Categorize your seniors

Not all seniors are the same. Grouping them helps you focus on what matters most for their age and stage. This is the system I created to help me quickly understand where my senior patients are in their aging journey and to help pet parents focus on what matters most for their dog at that stage. Please credit *The 3 Senior Dog Types™ Framework by Dr. Monica Tarantino, DVM* if you share or teach it.

3 Senior Dog Types™ Framework

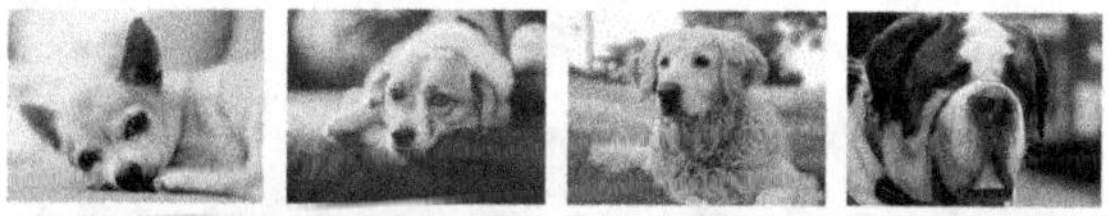

		0-20lbs	20-50lbs	50-80lbs	80+lbs+
Prevention of disease & delaying it	**Early Senior**	9-10 years	8-9 years	7-8 years	6-7 years
Disease Management & Prevention	**Classic Senior**	11-12 years	9-12 years	8-10 years	7-8 years
Quality of Life & Managing Disease	**Super Senior**	13-14+ years	11-12+ years	10-11+ years	9-10+ years

The 3 Senior Dog Types™ Framework was developed by Dr. Monica Tarantino, DVM, founder of the Senior Dog Veterinary Society. ©2025 Monica Tarantino. All rights reserved.

With each of the three types of senior dogs that walk through your clinic door, you will notice your conversations and medicine naturally shift toward two main areas, even though all areas remain important for every stage.

With **Early Seniors**, most of your focus will be on preventive medicine and client education, with a bit of early disease management sprinkled in.

With **Classic Seniors**, many of your discussions will revolve around disease management and ongoing prevention as conditions start to appear or progress.

And with **Geriatrics** or **Super Seniors**, your focus often shifts toward maintaining quality of life and managing chronic disease, while still addressing prevention through vaccines, dentals, and mobility maintenance.

New Vet Tip: I talk to owners a lot about their pets being *early seniors* because they often still look so good that owners don't believe they're seniors yet. This is actually the most critical time to start building awareness and helping them understand what they should be monitoring. The less time an owner spends in denial about their pet's age, the more proactive and realistic they become. Use these categories to guide your conversations and set expectations early.

5. Be a chronic pain champion

Every senior dog needs a chronic pain plan. Pain is one of the most common and most overlooked problems in older dogs. It's our job to manage it before it takes away quality of life.

The goal: institute a therapy plan that helps both prevent and reduce pain *to a level where it is well tolerated and does not interfere with daily activities or reduce quality of life* (AAHA, 2022).

Here's an example:

Becca: 14-year-old Lab mix with severe hip dysplasia confirmed on x-rays, moderate muscle wasting in both back legs and mild dental disease. Bloodwork over the past few years shows steadily increasing ALKP (now in 500's) on lab work. Weighs ~45lbs.

- Carprofen 75 mg PO q12h with food
- Joint diet and weight maintenance
- Movement plan: 3 short ½ to ¾ mile walks a day, PT to start in next month including underwater treadmill
- Contingency: add pregabalin 50–75 mg PO q8–12h or amantadine 100 mg q24h if pain worsens
- Recheck pain score in 4 weeks

This plan gives owners structure and confidence. One of my favorite anesthesiologists, Dr. Katie Bennett, always says every chronic pain plan should have a contingency. Owners love having a clear next step, and it keeps you proactive instead of reactive.

Chronic pain management is not a one-time plan, and owners need to understand that from the start. Follow up, reassess, and adjust regularly. Emphasize that you will be constantly tweaking and modifying the plan as their dog gets older or as chronic diseases progress. Check-ins and chats between the two of you will be really important as their pet ages.

If you want to dive deeper into pain management strategies, we have an excellent CE on chronic pain for SDVS members at www.seniordogvets.com.

Keep learning:

Interested in really honing your senior pet practice and taking your skills further? Check out the **Senior Dog Veterinary Society (SDVS)**- helping veterinarians everywhere give older dogs the life they deserve.

Here are a few easy ways to get started:

📋 **Senior Dog Wellness Screening Checklist**
Created by Dr. Monica Tarantino, DVM
Scan to download the one-page screening checklist I use in every senior appointment.

🎓 **Join our membership and get certified: Senior Dog Veterinary Society (Vet Students)**
Start your certification journey and build real confidence managing senior patients while still in school.

🐾 **Join our membership and get certified: Senior Dog Veterinary Society (Practicing Vets)**
Join the SDVS community and get certified in senior dog care.
Exclusive discount for *New Vet Jumpstart Guide* readers.

The 3 Senior Dog Types™ Framework was developed by Dr. Monica Tarantino, DVM, founder of the Senior Dog Veterinary Society. Used with permission.

NOTES:

NOTES:

CONCLUSION

This book has always been a passion project, born from the challenges, triumphs, and growth we experienced as early-career veterinarians. Now, with more years in the field and countless lessons collected along the way, our commitment to helping the next generation of veterinarians feels stronger than ever. The hurdles that shape your first year out are universal, and while there's no single path that makes the transition easy, there *are* tools, habits, and mindsets that make it manageable. Creating this book became our way of sharing these tools with you as your quick-reference companion that travels with you.

Your first year in practice will refine not just your medical knowledge and technical abilities, but your efficiency, communication, and confidence. It is a demanding season, and we built these cases to help lighten that load. Even though this edition highlights only a selection of cases, the way we walk you through them is meant to serve as a foundation you can apply universally. Our goal is to show you how seasoned veterinarians think and how we approach diagnostics, prioritize decisions, communicate effectively, build relationships, and keep patients moving forward. Over time, these thought processes become instinctive.

This book is now yours, so make it truly your own. Use the blank notes pages to capture pearls you learn from mentors, specialists, colleagues, conferences, and even your patients. Jot down client communication phrases that work well for you or save examples you may want to reference later. Think of this as both a guide and a growing archive of your evolving medical voice.

You will notice a major theme woven throughout these pages: great medicine requires great communication. Success in vet med doesn't come from diagnosing alone, it comes from guiding clients through understanding the disease, plan, treatment, and follow-up in a way they can truly grasp. A good veterinarian treats, while a great veterinarian teaches, supports, and builds trust. Remember: *clients only remember about 5% of what you tell them.* Let this set your expectations and shape your communication style.

A few reminders we stand by:

- **Chunk, then check in:** Share information in small, digestible pieces.
- **Pause for questions:** Let clients clarify along the way to avoid overwhelm.
- **Summarize simply:** Recap the key points and clearly outline the follow-up.
- **Send them home prepared:** Provide handouts, estimates, and written plans.
- **Follow up:** A call the next day can make all the difference.

As you grow, stay grounded in the truth that veterinary medicine is a lifelong journey. You will never stop learning...from textbooks, continuing education, specialists, and colleagues. Lean into mentorship, seek out diverse perspectives, uplift your peers, and contribute to the global community of veterinarians who strive every day to elevate our profession. We owe so much of this edition to the specialists and colleagues who generously shared their expertise in reviewing and refining these cases. Thank you for their time and dedication to mentorship. This book is stronger because of them.

And to those of you who are returning for the updated edition: thank you. Your support, loyalty, and passion for growth fuel everything we do.

We're grateful you're here. We're cheering for you, and we're committed to continuing this journey with you through future cases, our private podcast, monthly newsletters, and ongoing conversations on Instagram @vetsontherise and our website.

Now go take on this next chapter with confidence. You've got this, and we believe in you, every step of the way.

Your Vet Mentors,
Ashley and Monica

ABOUT THE AUTHORS

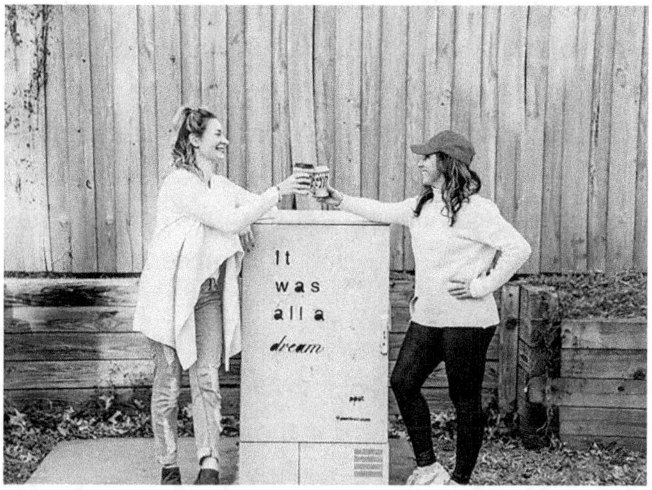

Ashley Gray and Monica Tarantino are two veterinarians united by a shared passion for guiding new graduates through the challenging, yet incredibly rewarding, transition into real-world practice. Both graduated from the Virginia-Maryland College of Veterinary Medicine in 2014 and began their careers in Charlotte, North Carolina. Ashley matched with a small animal rotating internship, while Monica stepped directly into a small animal general practice. Despite choosing different paths, they quickly discovered they were navigating many of the same obstacles that new grads still face today.

A year later, Ashley and Monica found themselves working side by side in a busy 24-hour hospital, where they mentored externs, interns, and early-career veterinarians. Those formative years were full of questions, late-night cases, growing pains, and shared breakthroughs. It revealed a truth that changed their careers: no new veterinarian is ever alone in their struggles. Every new grad faces similar challenges, and with the right support, guidance, and community, they can overcome them and thrive. That realization became the foundation of **VETS ON THE RISE**.

Today, Ashley and Monica continue to uplift the next generation of veterinarians, each while embracing new and deeply fulfilling chapters of their lives:

Monica Tarantino, DVM now practices part-time while growing her powerful movement dedicated to senior pet advocacy. Through **@seniordogdoc**, **@seniordogvets**, and the Senior Dog Revolution platform, Monica supports veterinarians and pet owners in improving the lives of senior dogs everywhere. Her passion for advancing senior care and educating the veterinary community has made her a trusted voice in this important niche of medicine.

Ashley Gray, DVM has transitioned into a part-time stay-at-home role, devoting her days to raising her two toddlers, supporting her husband, and caring for her lively crew of four senior pets. Alongside family life, she works in PR and social media, finding creativity and joy in a more flexible career chapter. After years of high-intensity leadership and clinical practice, Ashley has embraced this season as an opportunity to reset, heal, and focus intentionally on her mental health, an experience that continues to shape her compassion for veterinarians navigating their own life transitions. Follow along **@southernpetvet**

This second edition of their book is a testament to growth, both theirs and the Vet Med profession. Updated, expanded, and strengthened by invaluable input from veterinary specialists, it reflects their ongoing commitment to delivering the most relevant, practical, and supportive guidance for new veterinarians entering the field today.

With VETS ON THE RISE, Ashley and Monica remain dedicated to providing books, programs, tools, and community to help new grads rise with confidence, clarity, and connection in the amazing world of veterinary medicine.

VETS ON THE RISE

FOR STUDENTS & NEW GRAD VETS

Copyright 2026 by Dr. Ashley Gray and Dr. Monica Tarantino.
No portion of this book may be reproduced or transmitted in any form without prior written permission from the authors, except in the case of brief quotations published in articles and review.

NOTES:

NOTES:

www.ingramcontent.com/pod-product-compliance
Lightning Source LLC
LaVergne TN
LVHW080022210926
848481LV00011B/3085